Foreword from the Executive Director

AIDS is not over.
Together, we must overcome disruption and transform the AIDS response.

AIDS is not over—and this year's disruption to the global response has exposed the fragility of the progress we have fought so hard to achieve. Yet 2025 has also been a year of transformation, laying the foundations for a more sustainable, inclusive and nationally owned HIV response.

The impact of a sudden acceleration of cuts to international HIV financing, coupled with a retrenchment in human rights, has been devastating. The number of people using PrEP—HIV prevention medicines—has fallen by 64% in Burundi, 38% in Uganda and 21% in Viet Nam. Over 60% of all women-led HIV organizations have lost funding or been forced to suspend work, leaving entire communities without access to vital services.

A failure to reach the 2030 global HIV targets of the next Global AIDS Strategy could result in an additional 3.3 million new HIV infections between 2025 and 2030.

And yet we are seeing important signs of resilience. Communities are rallying to support each other and the AIDS response. Although the most impacted countries are also some of the most indebted, limiting their ability to invest in HIV, governments have taken swift action to increase domestic funding where they can. As a result, some countries have maintained or even increased the number of people receiving HIV treatment.

Regional initiatives such as the Accra Reset and the African Union Roadmap to 2030 and Beyond are carving out a new path towards health sovereignty. New agreements with generic pharmaceutical manufacturers will soon enable many developing countries to access long-acting injectable PrEP for just US$ 40 per person per year.

In a tough financial landscape, some donor governments are maintaining or increasing their commitment. The replenishment of the Global Fund to Fight AIDS, Tuberculosis and Malaria has so far secured pledges of more than US$ 11.34 billion.

World AIDS Day is a moment to renew our commitment to the AIDS response. In the hardest of circumstances, this is what I have seen this year—countries and communities coming together to overcome disruption and transform the response. It is within our grasp—we must seize it.

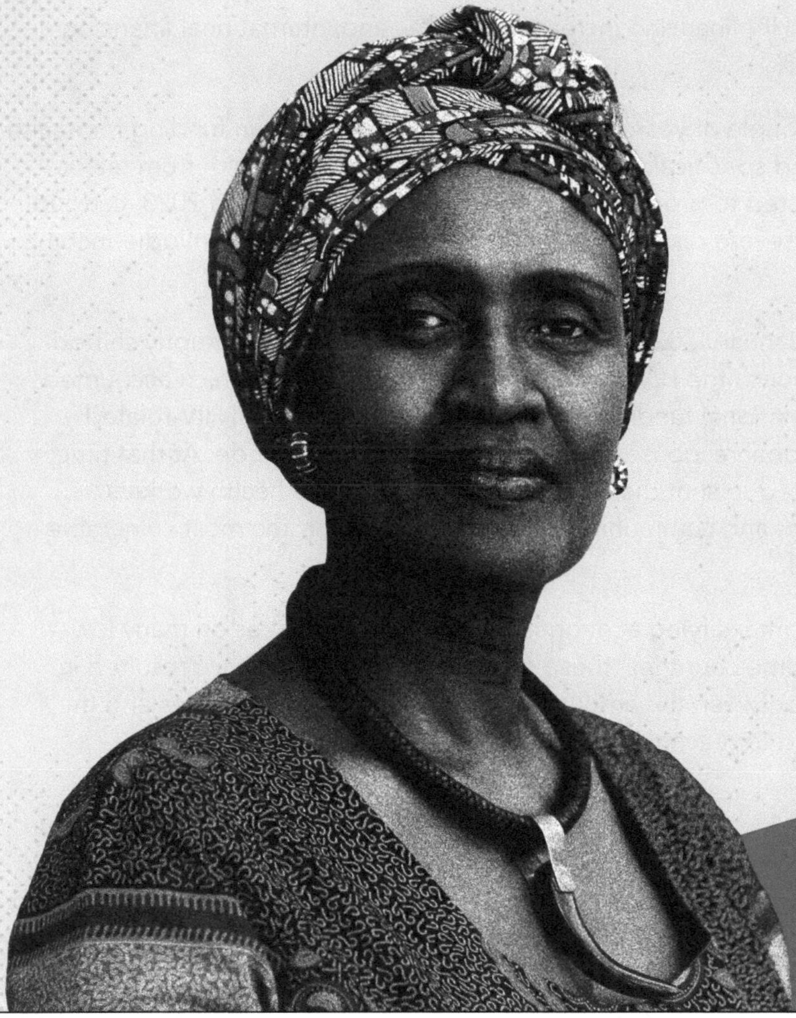

Winnie Byanyima
UNAIDS Executive Director

Introduction

At the end of 2024, the world was closer than in the past two decades to ending AIDS as a public health threat by 2030. At that point, 31.6 million of the 40.8 million (77%) [37 million–45.6 million] people living with HIV were on lifesaving treatment. HIV prevention and treatment services, and focusing on the societal barriers that put people at heightened risk of HIV, led to a 40% decrease in the number of new infections and a 54% decrease in the number of AIDS-related deaths between 2010 and 2024.

This progress was underpinned by a financing landscape that, although still not reaching the amounts needed to end AIDS, had shown global commitment from international donors and countries affected by HIV. Between 2010 and 2024, domestic HIV financing increased by 28%, and international financing increased by 12%.

Over the past couple of years, however, a remarkable drop in funding for health has occurred and specifically for HIV. International aid for health from major donors is projected to drop by 30–40% in 2025 compared with 2023, causing immediate and severe disruption to health services in low- and middle-income countries *(1)*.

Further, in late January 2025, the funding landscape for HIV abruptly shifted. The largest donor to the HIV response since the beginning, which accounted for 75% of international funding for HIV, temporarily halted all HIV-related funding. The global response immediately entered crisis mode. At that time, clinics were forced to shut their doors, essential frontline health workers were furloughed, and community programmes reaching the most vulnerable people stopped.

Combined with intensifying economic and financial pressures on many low- and middle-income countries, these collective funding cuts have resulted in a growing gap between the amounts available for HIV programmes and the amounts needed to reach the 2030 targets.

Even before the precipitous drop in funding in 2025, efforts to lay the foundation for a sustainable HIV response were uneven. Core components of long-term sustainability—preventing new HIV infections and maximizing viral load suppression among people living with HIV, which in turn prevent AIDS-related deaths and further HIV transmission—remained unachieved, with more than 11 million of the people living with HIV (27%) having an unsuppressed viral load in 2024.

Abrupt HIV funding reductions, persistent funding shortfalls and the perilous risks facing the global HIV response are having profound, lasting effects on the health and well-being of millions of people throughout the world. People living with HIV have died due to service disruptions, millions of people at high risk of acquiring HIV have lost access to the most effective prevention tools available, over 2 million adolescent girls and young women have been deprived of essential health services, and community-led organizations have been devastated, with many being forced to close their doors.

This report aims to capture the impacts of these disruptions, and the efforts countries and communities are making to overcome them and transform the HIV response to sustain the gains into the future. The impact has been most pronounced among lifesaving HIV prevention programmes and community organizations. The report also highlights examples of resilience from countries and communities to enable the response to move forward in the face of potentially existential threats.

Progress towards ending AIDS as a public health threat is real, but it remains fragile The decisions made in the coming weeks and months will determine whether the world ends AIDS by 2030 or whether the gains will be lost, numbers of new infections increase, and more people die from AIDS-related causes.

World AIDS Day 2025 offers an ideal moment for global reflection—on the massive progress made towards ending AIDS, on the new world order relating to HIV, and on the urgent need for solidarity and global commitment to end AIDS as a public health threat.

1

The HIV response is at risk

Progress in the global HIV response continued in 2024, although it was uneven and fell short of global AIDS 2025 and 2030 targets. The 1.3 million people newly acquiring HIV in 2024 was 40% lower than in 2010, and the number of AIDS-related deaths (630 000 in 2024) has continued to fall—by 54% since 2010 and by 15% since 2020.[1]

In 2024, antiretroviral therapy prevented 1.8 million [1.4 million–2.3 million] AIDS-related deaths. Over 30 million people have hope for a long, healthy future as a result of HIV prevention programmes. A recent study found that jurisdictions with higher coverage of pre-exposure prophylaxis (PrEP) have experienced markedly greater success in preventing new HIV acquisitions *(2)*.

Even before 2024, however, financial resources available for HIV programmes in low- and middle-income countries were well below the amounts needed to end AIDS as a public health threat (Figure 1.1). Over most of the past decade, HIV funding declined year on year, before a modest increase in 2024 *(3)*.

FIGURE 1.1

Estimated HIV resources available in low- and middle-income countries, 2010–2024 and projected need in 2030

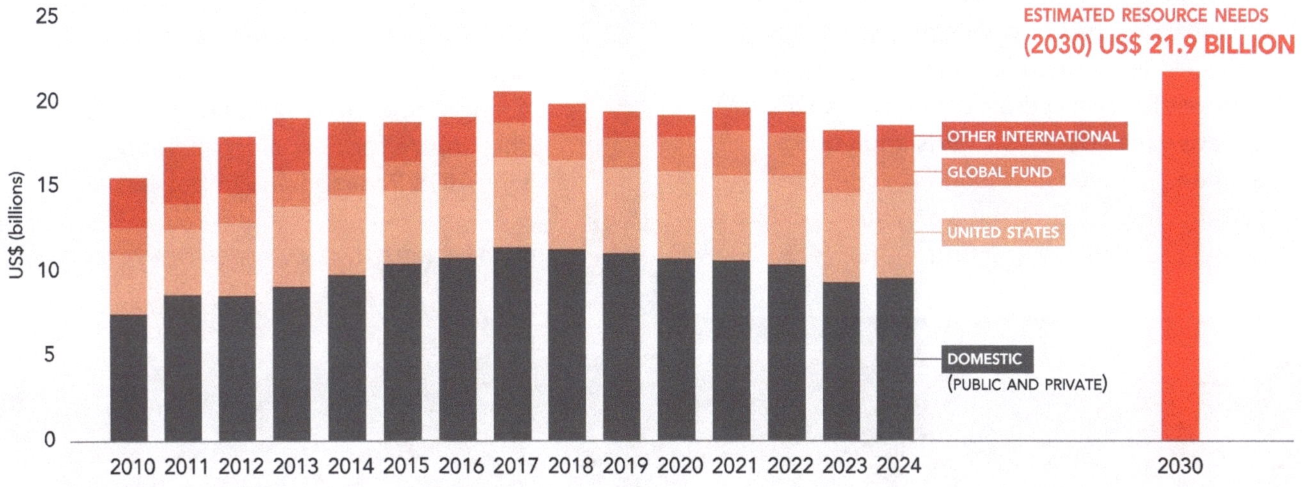

Note: low- and middle-income countries as per the World Bank income groups of countries, published July 2024.
Source: UNAIDS HIV financial estimates, July 2025.

Global declines in international health funding together with abrupt reductions in international HIV assistance in 2025 have deepened existing funding shortfalls. Although funding for some essential United States President's Emergency Plan for AIDS Relief (PEPFAR)-supported HIV programmes has restarted, service disruptions associated with these and other funding cuts are having long-lasting effects on almost all areas of the HIV response.

1 Unless otherwise indicated, all data cited in this report are available at https://aidsinfo.unaids.org. This includes monthly services delivery data under the Service Continuation tab.

The human impact of disruption

In 2025, the voices of people living with, at risk of or affected by HIV provide the most compelling evidence of the harms caused by the HIV funding crisis.[2]

"The only thing I could think of was my kids, and that I am going to die," says a South African sex worker aged 37 years and mother of three children, after losing access to antiretroviral therapy for four months *(4)*.

"It feels like the ground has been ripped out from under our feet. Before, we had places to go, people to talk to, and we knew someone cared. I felt supported when there were peer groups and community counsellors," says a woman living with HIV in Mozambique *(5)*.

"These [DREAMS] programmes empowered me and transformed my life," says Talent Manyoni, a young woman from Zimbabwe who lost access to accurate HIV information, sexual and reproductive health services, and educational and livelihood support following the closure of the DREAMS initiative for adolescent girls and young women. "I have witnessed firsthand the positive impact they have on young people's health, confidence and future prospects."

"The vulnerable populations we take care of do not trust our services any more. They say 'You went away without any notice and you were not available, you left us with nothing'," says Byrone Chingombe, Technical Director of the Centre for Sexual Health and HIV/AIDS Research in Zimbabwe.

2 Most of the following quotes are taken from interviews in October and November 2025 with people from community-led organizations to gather evidence of the impact of the funding cuts.

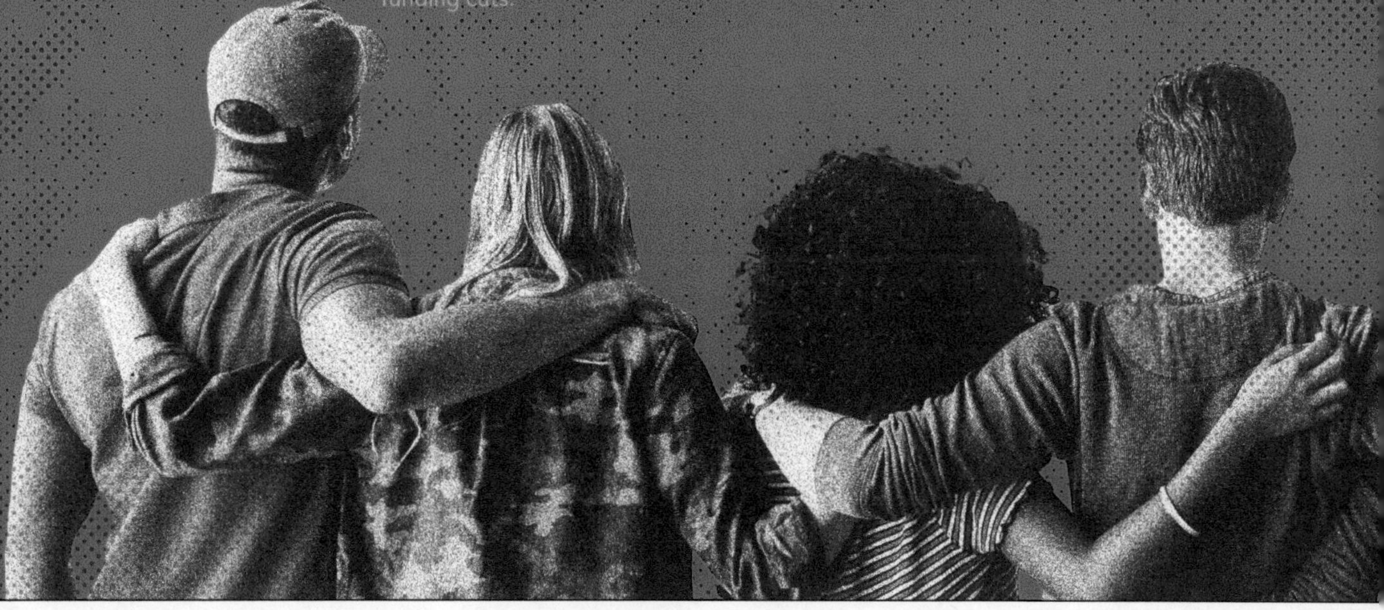

"[Funding cuts] created a situation where there is panic and an increase in mental health distress and anxiety," reports Jeffrey Walimbwa, Programmes Manager at Ishtar MSM, a Nairobi-based community-led organization in Kenya that serves gay men and other men who have sex with men. "There is a lot of fear because people are not sure what is happening."

"Social support networks of adolescent girls and young women have been weakened," says a peer educator in Uganda surveyed by the ATHENA Network. "Thousands of adolescent girls and young women are now isolated and detached from their networks ... The girls are scattered and this has increased their vulnerability" *(6)*.

"We have seen an increase in threats towards key populations," says Jeffrey Walimbwa of Ishtar MSM, in Kenya. "This is an attempt to erase our existence."

"In some countries, such as South Africa, where donor support for PrEP is now limited to pregnant and breastfeeding women, key population-focused PrEP programmes have been largely disintegrated," says Francois Venter of Ezintsha, South Africa.

"Community structures that supported people to remain engaged in care and come in for testing have been phased out," says Immaculate Bazare Owomugisha, Treasurer of the Global Executive Board of the International Community of Women Living with HIV based in Uganda. "The loss of funding forced the International Community of Women Living with HIV East Africa to lay off more than 30 people charged with conducting community-based monitoring."

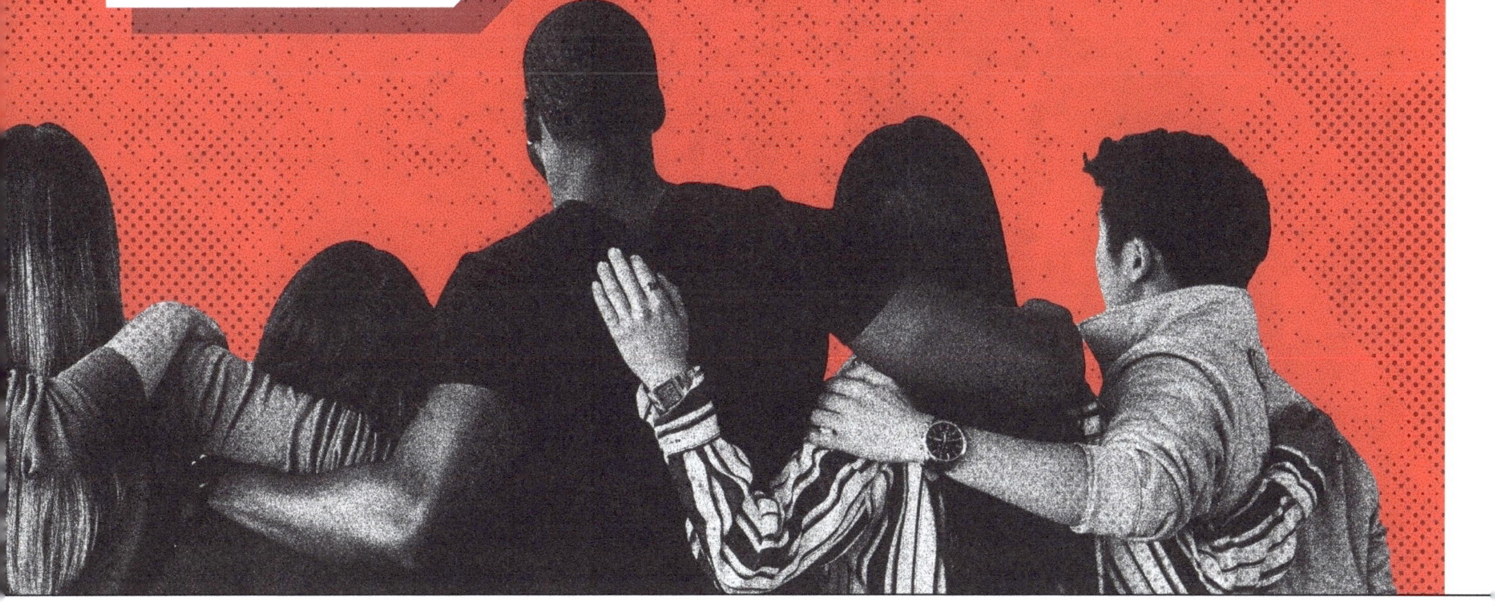

The challenges of monitoring the impact of HIV funding cuts in 2025

It is challenging to obtain up-to-the-minute data on the effects of funding cuts on people living with, at risk of or affected by HIV. Many countries report HIV service delivery data quarterly, resulting in time lags that make it difficult to obtain up-to-date understanding of a rapidly changing situation. The announcement of PEPFAR stop-work orders in early 2025 resulted in a flurry of rapid efforts to document and quantify service disruptions in the first part of 2025, but less information is available on the enduring effects on services in the latter half of the year.

Data monitoring in many countries has been curtailed due to cuts in funding because the data management staff were funded through the United States Government *(7)*. As a result, the number of service sites reporting data to national health authorities in 2025 varies within and between countries. Many community-led monitoring activities have been discontinued or reduced, undermining what has been an increasingly important source of person-centred data on the quality, reach and impact of services.

UNAIDS rapidly deployed the monthly Global AIDS Monitoring tool to work with countries to report on more real-time service delivery data through online reporting, but the quality and completeness of these data vary. Monthly reporting on disruptions and resumption of treatment services, for example, is available across 16 countries. Direct measures of the numbers of people acquiring HIV and AIDS-related deaths are difficult to produce for most countries. Modelled estimates compiled from countries and released by UNAIDS each year will be available only in July 2026 and will also come with uncertainty. This report aims to summarize the best available evidence regarding the impact of funding cuts on efforts to end AIDS as a public health threat, but the actual effects of funding cuts will likely become completely clear only over the next few years.

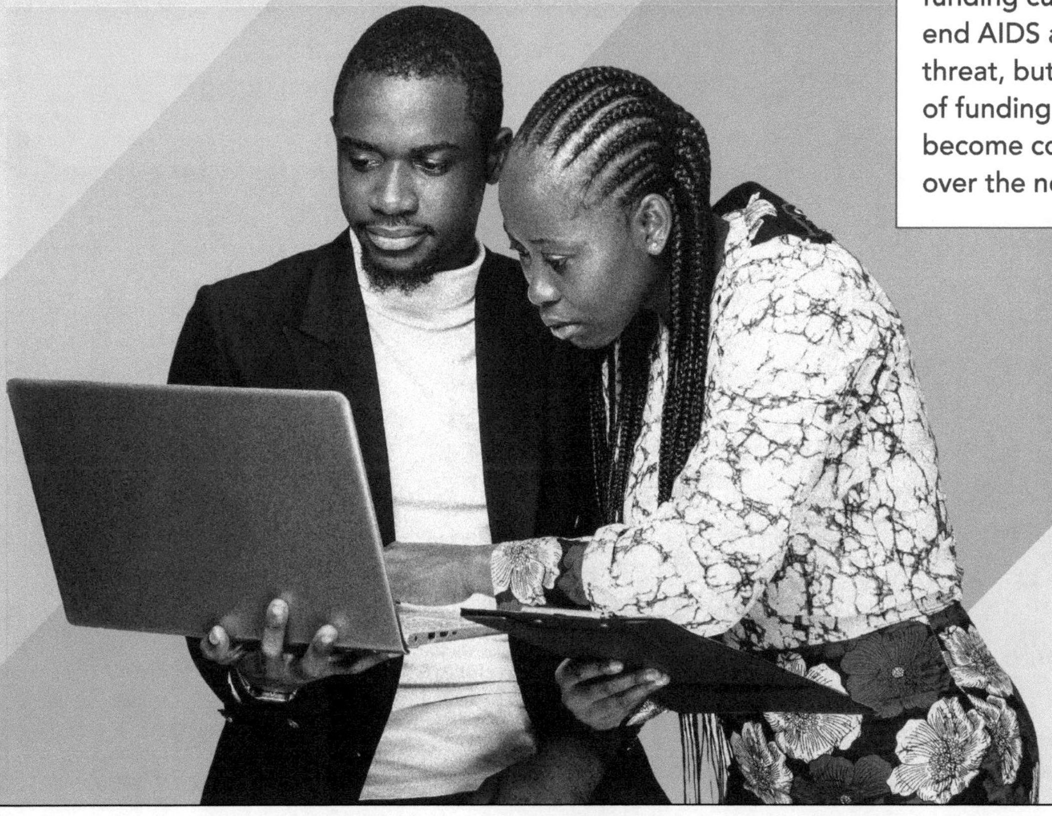

The vulnerability of the HIV response

Although the second part of 2025 has provided welcome signs of continued commitment from international donors to ending AIDS as a public health threat, including the United States of America, it is clear that the era of steady, year-on-year support through international HIV assistance is over. The Global Fund to Fight AIDS, Tuberculosis and Malaria (Global Fund) has identified more than 60 countries that might, in coming funding rounds, become ineligible for assistance or have their grants reduced, including a number of countries that have moved to upper-middle-income status in recent years *(8)*. The new United States America First Global Health Strategy provides significant funding and the ability to establish bilateral multiyear agreements that outline continued funding, co-investment on priority areas, and agreed upon transition trajectories for United States assistance, with increasing self-reliance for partner-country HIV responses by the end of these multiyear agreements *(9)*.

The most vulnerable aspects of the response persist, including HIV testing, prevention and care, data collection, community-led responses and community systems, human rights and gender equality programming, and enabling HIV services for people from key populations. Antiretroviral therapy programmes are largely financed domestically outside of sub-Saharan Africa, but such programmes are especially vulnerable to further donor reductions in western and central Africa, where donors provide 90% of treatment-related funding (including 53% provided by the Global Fund), and in eastern and southern Africa, where international support accounted for 38% of funding (Figure 1.2). For example, in Eswatini, where HIV prevalence is 23% among adults aged 15–49 years, the HIV programme lost 20% of its funding between 2024 and 2025, as a result of funding cuts from both bilateral and multilateral donors *(10)*.

FIGURE 1.2

External financing dependency by intervention and region, recent expenditure data, 2019–2024

	Eastern and southern Africa	Western and centralAfrica	Asia and the Pacific	Caribbean	Eastern Europe and central Asia	Latin America
Prevention	76% (16)	91% (12)	27% (16)	30% (2)	39% (11)	22% (11)
Condoms	33% (8)	44% (8)	17% (13)	12% (1)	62% (6)	5% (8)
HIV testing among key populations	81% (6)	100% (6)	6% (12)	70% (1)	60% (7)	75% (6)
Antiretroviral therapy	38% (7)	90% (8)	6% (12)	No data	7% (6)	1% (7)
Early infant diagnosis	2% (5)	100% (7)	32% (7)	No data	No data	50% (5)
Paediatric antiretroviral therapy	66% (7)	100% (7)	4% (8)	No data	64% (5)	3% (7)
Laboratory systems	20% (8)	98% (7)	8% (12)	17% (2)	12% (7)	9% (6)
Health systems strengthening	100% (8)	100% (7)	14% (9)	93% (1)	85% (5)	77% (6)
Strategic information	88% (7)	82% (6)	77% (10)	59% (1)	22% (5)	17% (6)

80–100% 60–<80% 40–<60% 20–<40% 0–<20% No data

Note: the number of countries (shown in parentheses) providing detailed granular expenditure data for each intervention varies across regions. As a result, the aggregate figures shown in the chart reflect only those countries that reported *(n)* such data for the respective intervention and region. The illustrated share of dependency is therefore influenced by the set of countries reporting in each region and may not represent all countries within the region. Following are the countries with usable data by region: **Asia and the Pacific:** Afghanistan, Bangladesh, Bhutan, Cambodia, India, Indonesia, Lao People's Democratic Republic, Malaysia, Mongolia, Nepal, Pakistan, Papua New Guinea, Philippines, Sri Lanka, Tajikistan, Thailand, Timor-Leste. **Caribbean:** Dominican Republic, Haiti. **Eastern and southern Africa:** Angola, Botswana, Comoros, Eritrea, Eswatini, Ethiopia, Kenya, Malawi, Mozambique, Namibia, Rwanda, South Africa, Uganda, United Republic of Tanzania, Zambia, Zimbabwe. **Eastern Europe and central Asia:** Albania, Armenia, Azerbaijan, Belarus, Georgia, Kazakhstan, Kyrgyzstan, North Macedonia, Republic of Moldova, Ukraine, Uzbekistan. **Latin America:** Belize, Brazil, Colombia, Costa Rica, Ecuador, El Salvador, Guatemala, Honduras, Paraguay, Peru, Venezuela (Bolivarian Republic of). **Middle East and North Africa:** excluded from this analysis because there were no recent granular expenditure data for each of the intervention areas. **Western and central Africa:** Benin, Burkina Faso, Central African Republic, Chad, Democratic Republic of the Congo, Gabon, Gambia, Ghana, Guinea, Mali, Nigeria, Senegal, Togo.

Figures on health systems strengthening reflect lower level of granular data reported from countries. It includes activities related to health sector governance and planning, community system support, public financial management systems, and workforce development and quality improvement.It excludes other aspects of health systems such as lab management and strategic information which are shown separately.

Source: Global AIDS Monitoring, UNAIDS-supported national AIDS spending assessments, 2019–2024.

Other aspects of the response are also at risk. For example, countries in western and central Africa, where numbers of new HIV infections have not declined and where 1.3 million of the 5.2 million people living with HIV are not on treatment, depend on external donors for 99% of laboratory funding. Laboratory services are critical to the HIV response, enabling prompt HIV diagnosis and linkage to care, informing clinical decision-making on switching regimens, and aiding management of advanced HIV disease.

Risks to HIV prevention efforts

FIGURE 1.3

Funding for HIV prevention programmes by region, 2019–2024

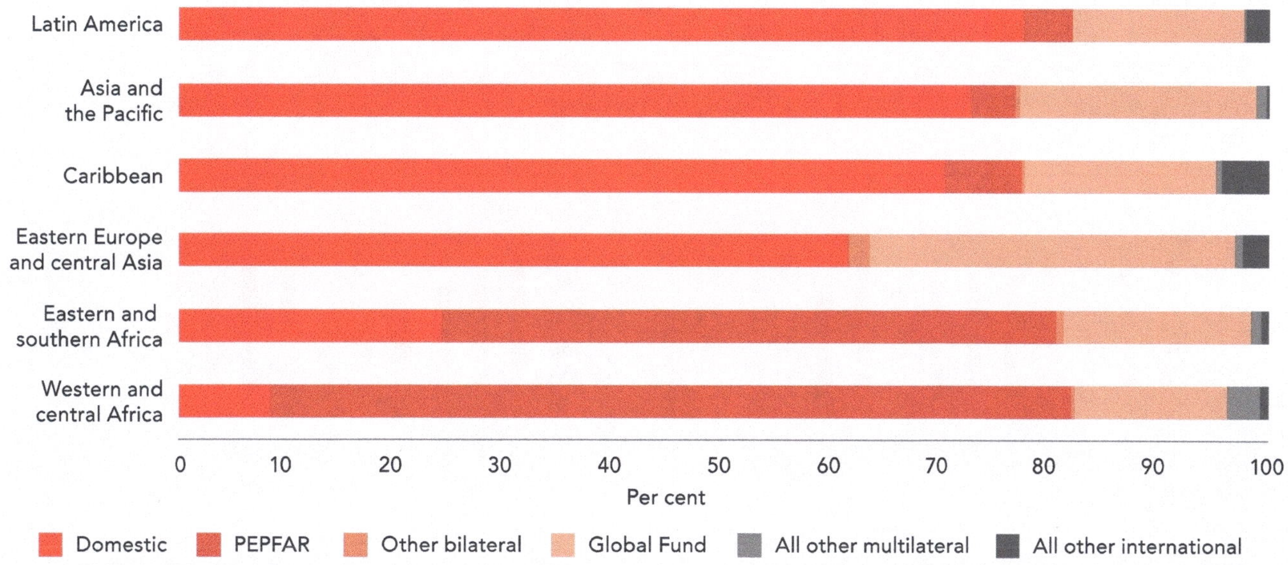

Note: the Middle East and North Africa did not have granular data for this intervention, and therefore it is not included. Asia and the Pacific region (all GAM-reporting countries) relies on international funding for 27% of HIV prevention resources overall. This rises to 55% when India is excluded, underscoring the region's particularly high dependence on international sources.
Source: Global AIDS Monitoring, UNAIDS-supported national AIDS spending assessments, 2019–2024.

Lack of domestic funding for prevention programmes coupled with declines in donor HIV assistance for such programmes has devastated HIV prevention services, which historically have relied heavily on donor assistance in most regions, with especially high donor dependency in sub-Saharan Africa (Figure 1.3). This is in contrast to HIV testing and treatment services, for which access declined but has now rebounded in many countries since the funding cuts.

Funding cuts have substantially affected access to PrEP. As of 15 October 2025, the AIDS Vaccine Advocacy Coalition estimates that 2.5 million people who used PrEP in 2024 lost access to their medicines in 2025 due to donor cuts *(11)*. Effects are apparent in diverse countries, with a 31% decline in the number of people receiving PrEP in Uganda from December 2024 to September 2025, 21% decline in Viet Nam from December 2024 to June 2025 (Figure 1.5), 23% over the first eight months of 2025 in Ukraine, and 64% from December 2024 to August 2025 in Burundi. In a few countries (e.g. Cambodia, Ghana, Lao People's Democratic Republic, Mozambique), there is some evidence that PrEP uptake has recovered somewhat following earlier service disruptions.

Funding disruptions imperil future progress towards eliminating new HIV infections among children. In Ghana, where 1200 (850–2300) children acquired HIV in 2024, the number of pregnant women living with HIV who delivered during the past month and received antiretroviral medicines for their own health and to prevent HIV transmission to their children fell by 29% during the first six months of 2025 (Figure 1.4). Across sub-Saharan Africa, 450 000 people have lost access to mother2mother mentors—peer educators who council and support pregnant women and new mothers—and other health services critical for their own health and the prevention of new HIV acquisition among children *(12)*.

FIGURE 1.4

Number of pregnant women living with HIV who delivered during the past month and received antiretroviral medicines to reduce the risk of vertical transmission of HIV, October 2024 to October 2025

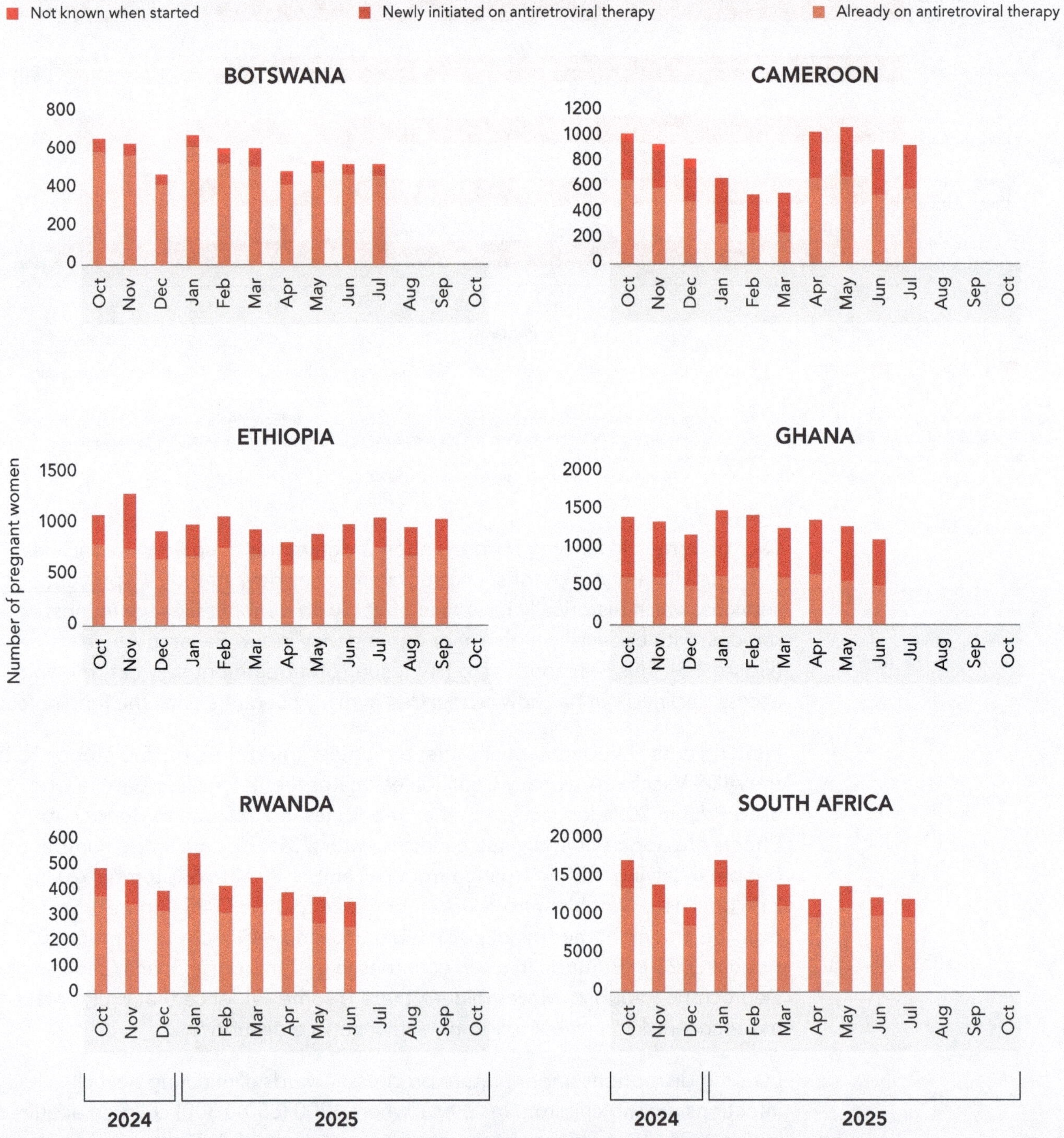

Source: country-reported data through the monthly Global AIDS Monitoring platform (https://aidsinfo.unaids.org/services).

Access to proven HIV combination prevention tools is declining at the very moment when demand should be expanding, especially as innovations are coming on to the market, including long-acting injectable PrEP. Between December 2024 and March 2025, the number of male condoms distributed fell by 55% in Nigeria, with more modest reductions reported in Uganda. As recently as October 2025, Botswana was reportedly experiencing widespread shortages of HIV test kits, condoms and treatments for sexually transmitted infections *(13)*.

Access to voluntary medical male circumcision, which reduces the risk of female-to-male sexual transmission by about 60% *(14)* and offers comparable protection to men who have sex with men *(15)*, has declined due to funding cuts. The number of voluntary medical male circumcisions fell by 65% in Uganda between December 2024 and June 2025 and by 88% in Botswana during the first five months of 2025, although uptake has rebounded more recently in some countries, such as Lesotho and Malawi.

RISKS TO HIV PREVENTION FOR ADOLESCENT GIRLS, YOUNG WOMEN AND SURVIVORS OF GENDER-BASED VIOLENCE

Adolescent girls and young women represent 25% of all new HIV acquisitions in sub-Saharan Africa.

The total number of adolescent girls and young women aged 15–24 years acquiring HIV has fallen by half globally since 2010, and by a similar margin in eastern and southern Africa and western and central Africa. These declines generally align with levels of access to effective HIV treatment. Although progress has been achieved in reducing the number of new HIV infections among women and girls since 2010, young women and girls continue to be disproportionately affected by HIV in sub-Saharan Africa. Since 2010, new HIV infections have declined by 62% among boys aged 15–24 years but by only 51% among adolescent girls and young women. **There were 570 new HIV infections among adolescent girls and young women globally a day in 2024.**

Reductions in donor assistance had especially acute effects on efforts to prevent new HIV infections among adolescent girls and young women, especially through the DREAMS initiative, a comprehensive multisectoral package of biomedical, behavioural and structural interventions and services for the most vulnerable adolescent girls and young women in 15 high-burden countries. Among 444 adolescent girls and young women surveyed in 2025 by the ATHENA Network and UNAIDS across 10 countries in sub-Saharan Africa, 48% reported that their communities had experienced disruptions with respect to access to services for HIV prevention and treatment and sexual and reproductive health *(6)*. At one programme in Kenya, that supported 66 000 adolescent girls and young women who remained HIV-free after three years of DREAMS services, a young woman reported feeling "hopeless" after the programme was abruptly halted, with many service recipients now forced to live in cramped shelters and depend on charitable donations *(16)*.

Funding cuts are depriving survivors of sexual violence of the services they need. According to Physicians for Human Rights, services for survivors of sexual violence, including post-exposure HIV prophylaxis (medicine taken in the 48 hours after sex to prevent HIV acquisition), declined in the Democratic Republic of the Congo as a result of the cuts *(17)*. In Ethiopia, funding cuts have prompted providers to impose out-of-pocket user fees for post-exposure HIV prophylaxis services for survivors of rape, which previously were delivered free of charge *(18)*.

RISKS TO HIV RESPONSES FOR KEY POPULATIONS

Programmes serving vulnerable populations are essential to reduce new HIV infections and accelerate progress towards ending AIDS as a public health threat. Donor funding accounts for most of the funding (100% in western and central Africa) for tailored HIV testing services in settings focusing on key populations, including gay men and other men who have sex with men, sex workers, people who inject drugs, transgender people, gay men and other men, people in prisons and other closed settings, and adolescent girls and young women. Available evidence indicates that key populations experience below-average coverage for HIV treatment and prevention services, with prevention services currently reaching less than 50% of people from these populations *(19)*.

FIGURE 1.5

Number of people who receieved pre-exposure prophylaxis (PrEP) at least once during the reporting period, monthly, October 2024 to October 2025

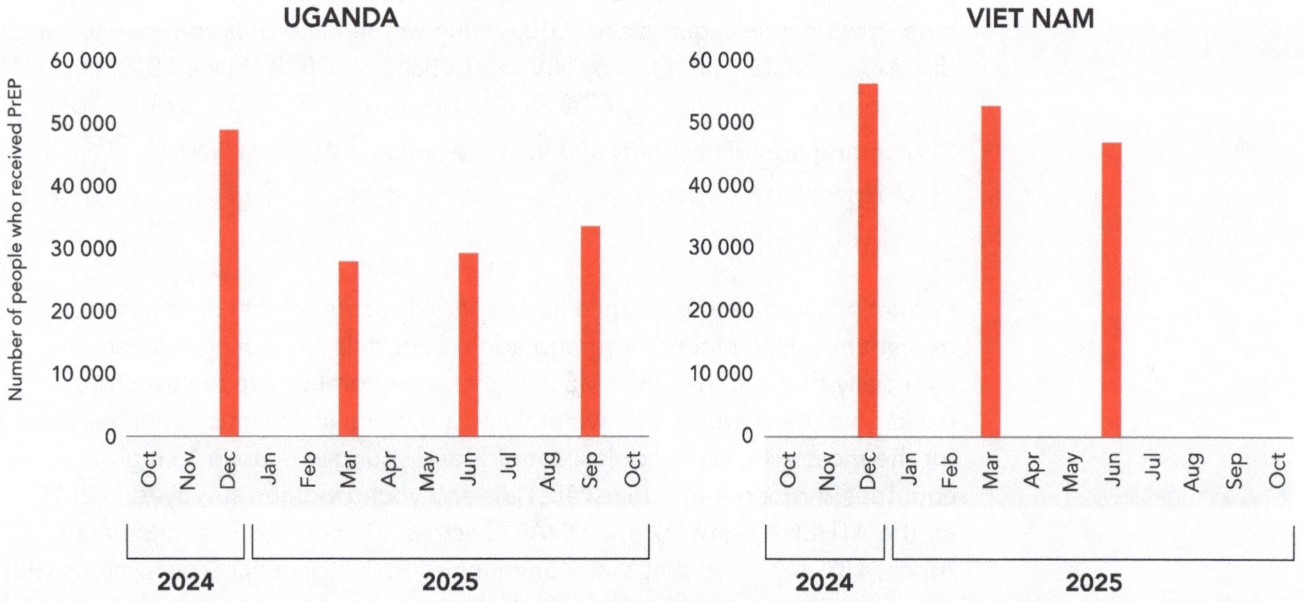

Source: country-reported data through the monthly Global AIDS Monitoring platform (https://aidsinfo.unaids.org/services).

The reduction in donor HIV financing in 2025 has deeply undermined efforts to address the HIV-related needs of people from key populations. In some countries, such as Zimbabwe, many HIV services for sex workers and other people from key populations have effectively collapsed in 2025 because of funding cuts *(20)*. Cessation of donor support for population-focused HIV prevention services led to the termination of most drop-in clinics for people from key populations in Kenya, the closure of at least five clinics for people from key populations in Nigeria, and the partial or full closure of 45% of HIV programmes serving people from key populations in Uganda *(21)*. In April 2025, an online survey found that 77% of harm reduction programmes and other HIV services for people who inject drugs had been severely disrupted by funding cuts *(22)*.[3] Reports from UNAIDS country offices demonstrate a marked rollback in HIV prevention services in prisons and other closed settings. In some countries, such as Kenya, where PEPFAR support for PrEP is now limited to pregnant and breastfeeding women, key population-focused PrEP programmes have stopped *(24)*. The sharp funding cuts for key population programmes have been accompanied by increases in hostile attacks and harassment towards people from key populations in many countries *(21)*.

Alarmingly, these service disruptions are occurring at a time when the proportion of new HIV infections among some key populations is rising. Analysis by UNAIDS to model the estimated incidence among key populations between 2010 and 2024 found that, globally, the share of new HIV infections among people from key populations and their partners rose from 44% in 2010 to 49% in 2024 (Figure 1.6).

FIGURE 1.6

Trends in numbers of new adult HIV infections by population, global, 2010–2024

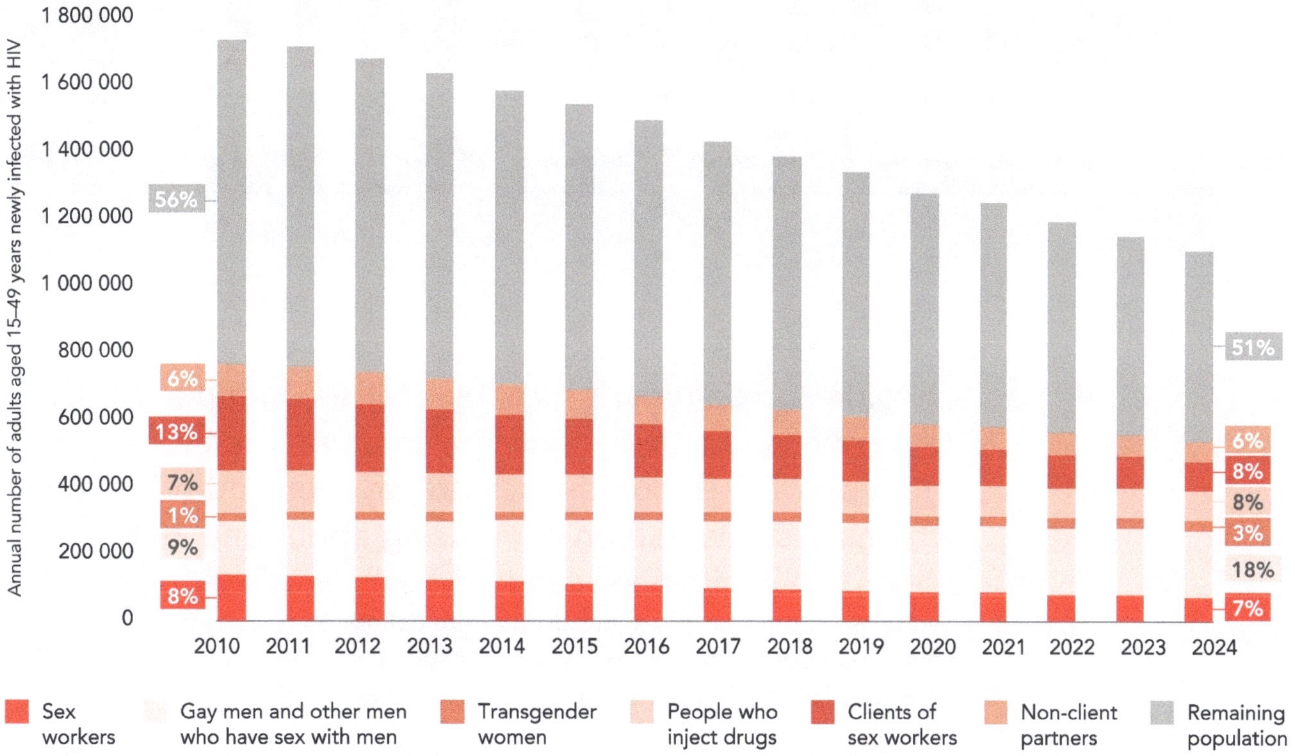

Source: UNAIDS special analyses, 2025.

3 Harm reduction is a "set of policies, programmes, services and actions that aim to reduce the harm to individuals, communities and society related to drugs, including HIV infection". For more information on the services included in the comprehensive harm reduction package, see the WHO Policy Guidance by HIV Intervention Area *(23)*.

These new UNAIDS estimates show substantial variation between regions. Within sub-Saharan Africa, heterosexual transmission continues to predominate, with people from populations not classified as key populations or their sexual partners accounting for 74% of new HIV infections in 2024 (Figure 1.7).

FIGURE 1.7
Trends in numbers of new adult HIV infections by population, sub-Saharan Africa, 2010–2024

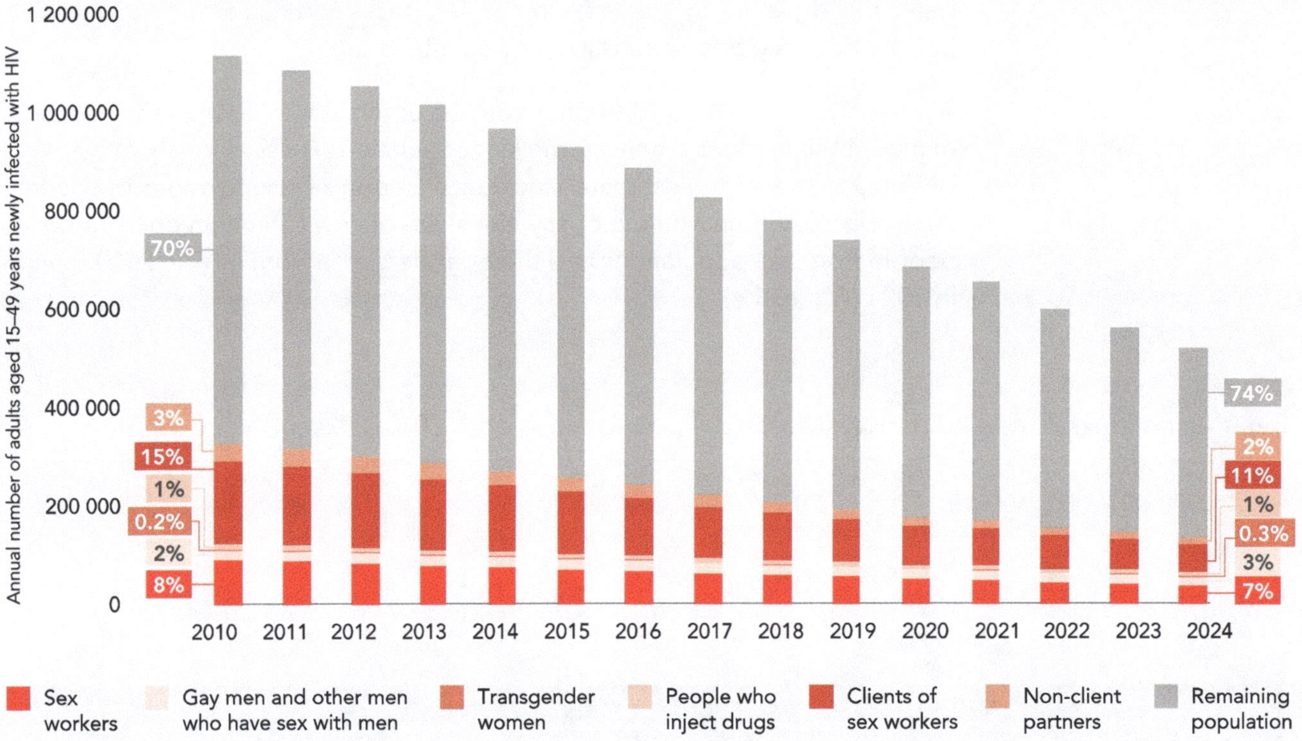

Source: UNAIDS special analyses, 2025.

Outside sub-Saharan Africa, by contrast, people from key populations and their sexual partners account for two in three new HIV acquisitions, with gay men and other men who have sex with men comprising about one in three adults (31%) with newly acquired HIV. In eastern Europe and central Asia, people who inject drugs were estimated to constitute the largest annual number of people from key populations with newly acquired HIV—25% of all new infection regionally in 2024 (Figure 1.8).

FIGURE 1.8

Trends in numbers of new adult HIV infections by population, outside sub-Saharan Africa, 2010–2024

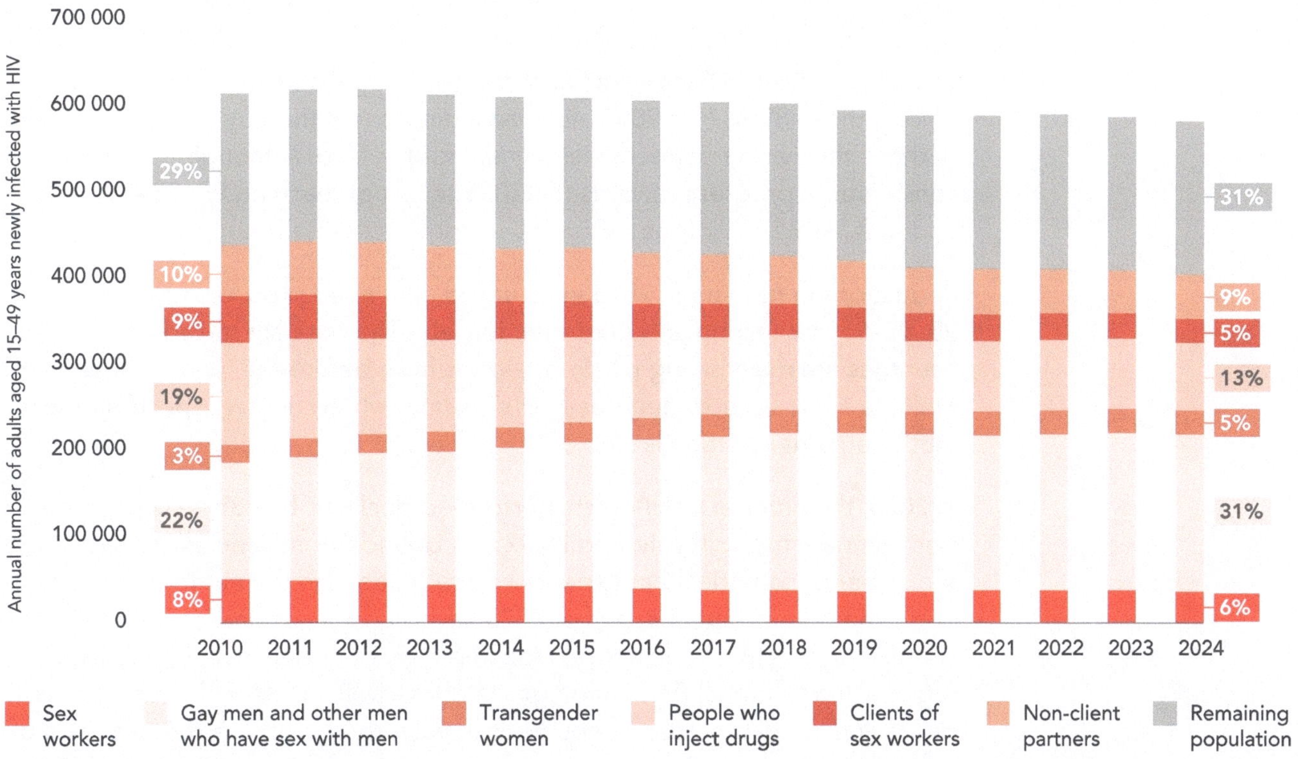

Source: UNAIDS special analyses, 2025.

Globally, the annual number of new adult HIV acquisitions overall has declined steadily (by 36%) since 2010. From 2010 to 2024, however, the number of new adult HIV acquisitions increased by 27% among gay men and other men who have sex with men and by 32% among transgender women. For both of these key populations, their share of new HIV acquisitions rose two-fold between 2010 and 2024 (Figure 1.6). The number of new HIV infections declined among sex workers (by 48%), people who inject drugs (by 33%) and clients of sex workers (by 61%) between 2010 and 2024, due in large measure to the success of HIV prevention efforts among these key populations.

Risks to HIV testing and treatment services

Globally, in 2024, 87% [69–>98%] of people living with HIV knew their status, among those 89% [71–>98%] received antiretroviral therapy and 94% (75–>98%] of those receiving treatment were virally suppressed. Although this shows the considerable progress towards the 2025 target of reaching 95–95–95, at the end of 2024 9.2 million people were still not accessing treatment *(7)*.[4]

Reductions in funding in 2025 interrupted continued progress towards the 95–95–95 HIV testing and treatment targets. The data are mixed on whether countries are maintaining treatment levels from before the funding cuts. Multiple sources show declines in HIV testing, while country reports suggest that treatment initiation is stable.

In 2025, the number of HIV tests performed declined by 43% in Cameroon from January through July, and by 17% in Uganda from January through June. A number of countries that experienced reductions in the number of HIV tests performed during the first half of 2025 have managed more recently to increase HIV testing (e.g. Burundi, Kenya, Mozambique, Rwanda). In an unpublished regional International Epidemiology Database to Evaluate AIDS survey of HIV clinics and cohorts across 32 countries in eastern and southern Africa, 24% of respondents reported interruptions in access to early infant diagnosis from January to July 2025.

Compared with the last quarter of 2024, numbers of people initiated on antiretroviral therapy in the first three months of 2025 dropped between 2% and 22% across the 13 countries in sub-Saharan Africa and south-east Asia for which data are available *(25)*. Countries reporting to UNAIDS have reported relatively steady numbers or even an increase in new initiations on antiretroviral therapy (Figure 1.9), but the quality of those continuing services might be of lower. Community-led monitoring conducted by Ritshidze documented a "system-wide slide" in HIV clinical service delivery across South Africa, with 48% of public health clinics reporting a lasting negative impact of funding disruptions on clinic capacity, including increased waiting times and staffing shortages *(26)*. Months after the initial PEPFAR stop-work order, 71% of 34 health-care facilities surveyed in Zambia reported persistent negative effects on clinic capacity, including staff shortages, delays in providing services, and shortages of diagnostics and other laboratory services *(27)*.

4 The targets call for 95% of all people living with HIV to know their HIV status, 95% of all people diagnosed with HIV to receive antiretroviral therapy, and 95% of all people receiving antiretroviral therapy to have a suppressed viral load by 2025.

FIGURE 1.9

Number of new antiretroviral therapy initiations, October 2024 to October 2025

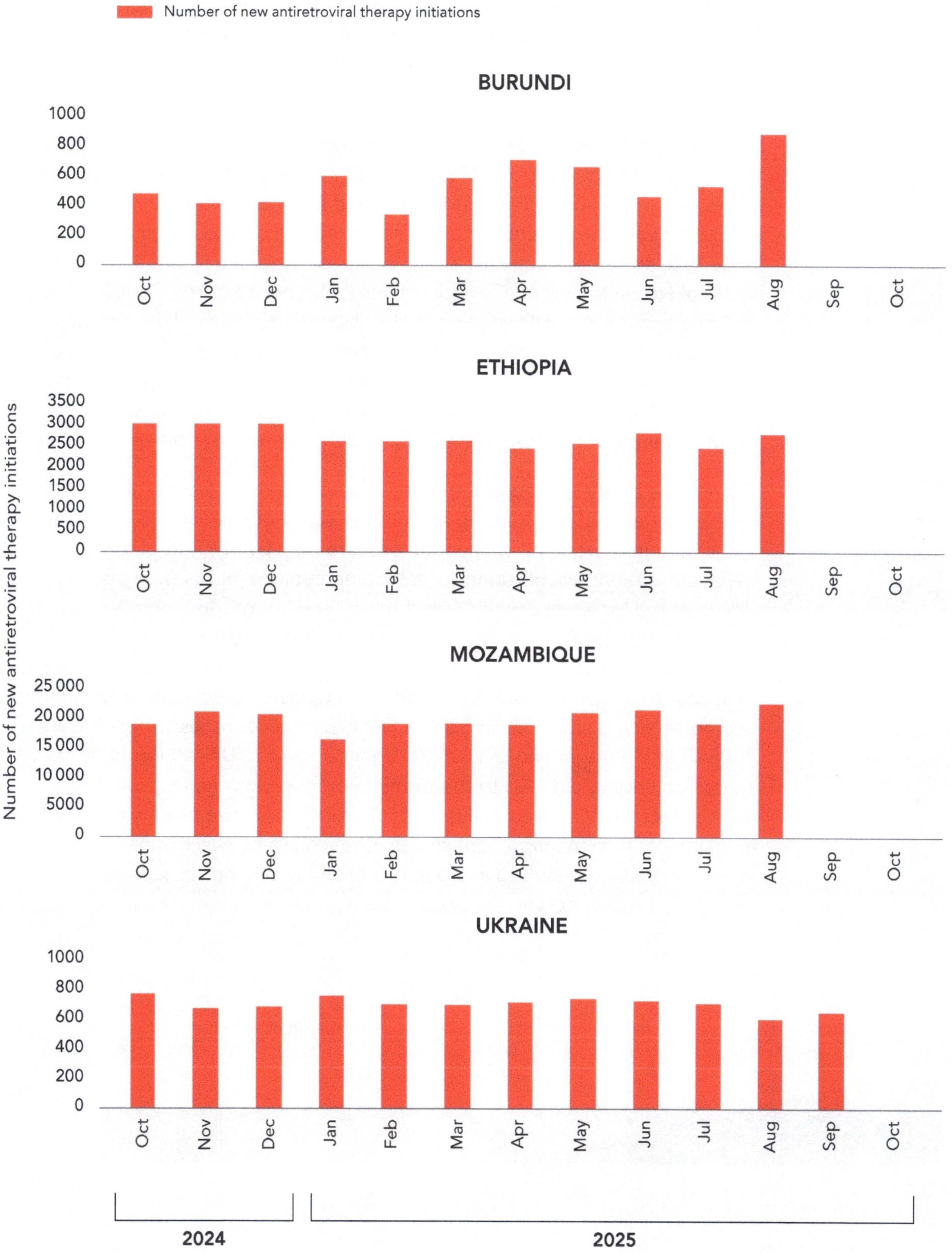

Source: country-reported data through monthly Global AIDS Monitoring platform (https://aidsinfo.unaids.org/services).

Funding shortfalls in 2025 have disrupted access to essential viral load monitoring in many settings. A survey by the Clinton Health Access Initiative (CHAI) found that the number of viral load tests performed fell by 16–68% across 13 countries *(23)*. In an unpublished International Epidemiology Databases to Evaluate AIDS survey among 68 HIV clinics and eight programmatic cohorts in Asia and the Pacific, eastern and southern Africa and Latin America, 24% of respondents reported disruptions to access viral load testing during the first seven months of 2025.

Declines in the number of CD4 tests performed from the last quarter of 2024 to the first quarter of 2025 in countries surveyed by CHAI varied from 3% to 64% *(25)*. Reduced access to viral load and CD4 count monitoring, combined with the potentially diminished ability of HIV programmes to undertake adherence support and client re-engagement functions due to financial stresses, potentially undermines the capacity of HIV clinics to identify and manage people with advanced HIV disease. Advanced HIV disease, which persists as a major barrier to optimizing the public health impact of antiretroviral therapy *(28)*, is closely linked with access to and uptake of HIV testing and antiretroviral therapy, CD4 testing, treatment adherence and prompt re-initiation for people who have dropped out of care *(29)*.

Disruptions in HIV testing and treatment services in 2025 stemmed from many different effects of HIV funding reductions. Many of the over 350 000 health and community workers whose salaries were paid by PEPFAR globally *(9)* were temporarily laid off during the funding cuts earlier in 2025, resulting in documented losses of essential health worker positions in countries such as Kenya *(30)* and Zambia *(27)*. Many clinics funded through external assistance either shut down earlier this year or curtailed their services, with an unpublished multicountry International Epidemiology Databases to Evaluate AIDS survey finding service disruptions at 53% of HIV clinics in countries supported by PEPFAR at the beginning of 2025. In Uganda and the United Republic of Tanzania, funding cuts led to the termination of programmes providing differentiated HIV service delivery *(31)*. Disruptions in commodity procurement and supply-chain management systems, which are heavily donor-dependent in many countries, resulted in stockouts of HIV medicines in several settings, including the Democratic Republic of the Congo *(17)*, Ethiopia *(18)* and Kenya *(30)*.

Risks to community-led responses

Cuts in international HIV assistance are having especially ruinous consequences for community-led services, which often depend wholly on external assistance. Data from eight countries that have recently undertaken national AIDS spending assessments (Bangladesh, Belize, Benin, Côte d'Ivoire, Mozambique, Nigeria, Pakistan, Papua New Guinea) indicate that community-led organizations rely on bilateral partners for 89% and multilateral donors for 10.9% of their funding, with less than 0.1% of operating support coming from domestic sources *(32)*.

Funding uncertainties are already jeopardizing community-led responses across the world. Community-led organizations of gay men and other men who have sex with men in Kenya, Mozambique and Viet Nam have been forced by the discontinuation of donor funding to reduce staffing, with layoffs ranging from a third of organizational staff to nearly all clinical staff (personal communication, A Spieldenner, MPACT, 8 October 2025). Community outreach services have been reduced or eliminated altogether in Angola and Eswatini due to funding cuts *(33)*. Over 60% of women-led HIV organizations have lost funding or been forced to suspend essential programmes, leaving entire communities without access to vital services *(34)*. A survey of 45 youth-led and youth-serving organizations, 56% of which are based in sub-Saharan Africa, revealed that 60% had experienced a sudden and significant loss of resources *(35)*.

The contributions of community-led organizations to national HIV responses are wide-ranging. They include substantial delivery of HIV prevention, testing, care and treatment services; interventions for social protection and economic support; systems strengthening and societal enablers; and preventing and responding to gender-based violence. In countries reporting these data to UNAIDS, more than 80% of sex workers, gay men and other men who have sex with men, and transgender people relied on nongovernmental organizations, including those led by people from key populations, for condoms and lubricants (Figure 1.10). For people who inject drugs, the public sector was a minor source of needles and syringes but the largest provider of opioid agonist maintenance therapy (Figure 1.10).

FIGURE 1.10

Distribution of reported services for people from key populations, by type of provider, 2020–2024

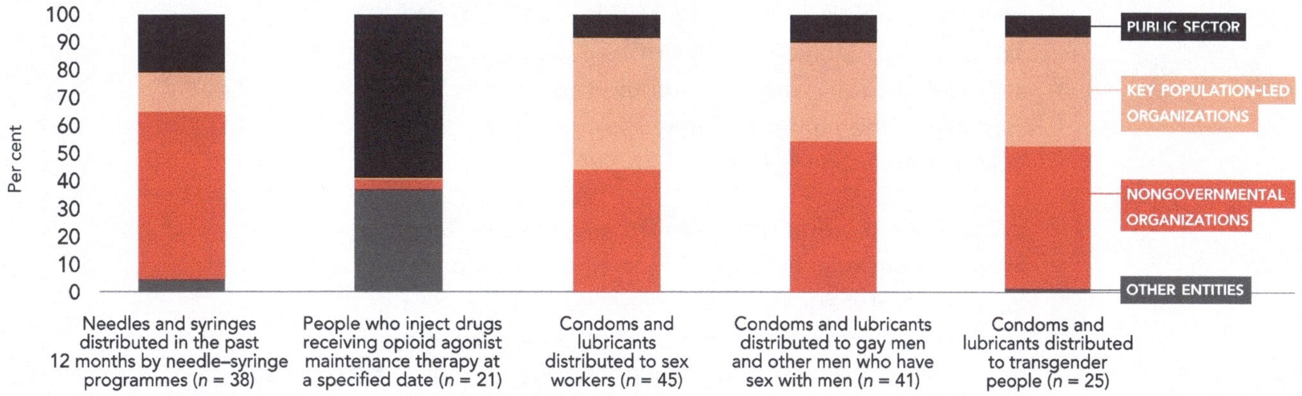

Note: *n* = number of countries.
Source: Global AIDS Monitoring, 2021–2025 (https://aidsinfo.unaids.org/)

The impact of donor cuts on community-led responses in Tajikistan

Takhmina Haidarova and Pulod Jamalov are among the very few HIV activists in Tajikistan living openly with HIV. For years, they have been the public faces of courage—challenging stigma, supporting other people and ensuring no one faces HIV alone. Through their organizations, the Tajikistan Network of Women Living with HIV and Spin Plus, they have built lifelines for people living with HIV and people from key populations, including people who use drugs.

Now those lifelines are at risk of disappearing. Funding freezes and cuts to international HIV assistance threaten to close community-led programmes across the country. "People are panicking," says Takhmina. "If our support services shut down, women affected by HIV, families with children living with HIV, and people from key populations will have nowhere to turn."

Across Tajikistan, nearly 97% of women living with HIV conceal their HIV status, even from family members, and 64% report discrimination, including from health-care providers.

"Community groups like ours are the only ones people trust," says Pulod Jamalov, Director of Spin Plus. "We go where the system does not reach—into prisons, remote villages and migrant families. Without us, many people will simply be left behind."

Although HIV-related mortality has halved since 2020, progress is fragile. About 60% of the HIV response in Tajikistan still depends on international donors, of which 20% was funded by PEPFAR until January 2025. National authorities estimate that even a 10–20% funding reduction could trigger a 135% increase in the number of new HIV infections and a 5% increase in mortality—erasing years of gains.

In 2025, for the first time, the Government of Tajikistan allocated national funds to procure 10% of the country's antiretroviral medicines. Tajikistan has shown what is possible with targeted support. But unless donors, governments and international partners act quickly to protect community-led services, those gains will be reversed.

A growing human rights crisis

There are signs that the global climate for human rights and gender equality is worsening, exacerbating the harms from HIV funding cuts *(36, 37)*, with especially severe consequences for marginalized populations. In 2025, for the first time since UNAIDS began monitoring punitive laws in 2008, the number of countries criminalizing same-sex sexual activity and gender expression increased. Globally, anti-gender and anti-rights movements are growing in influence and geographic reach, jeopardizing gains made to date on the rights of women and girls, people living with HIV and LGBTIQ+ people *(38)*.

Currently, in 2025, 168 countries criminalize some aspect of sex work, 152 impose criminal penalties for the possession of small amounts of drugs, 64 criminalize same-sex relations and 14 criminalize transgender people. Cases of criminal prosecution of people living with HIV are on the rise, and 48 new HIV-related criminal cases were reported across 23 countries between January and June 2025 *(39)*.[5] People living with HIV are vulnerable to criminal prosecution in 156 countries for HIV nondisclosure, exposure or transmission, even though experts agree these laws are scientifically groundless and ineffective in preventing HIV transmission (Figure 1.11). Punitive laws slow uptake of HIV testing, disclosure and treatment, with a study in western and central Africa finding that "sex workers and women living with HIV avoid health facilities for fear of denunciation or arrest" *(40)*.

FIGURE 1.11

Countries with laws criminalizing HIV nondisclosure, exposure or transmission or prosecutions based on general criminal laws, global, 2025

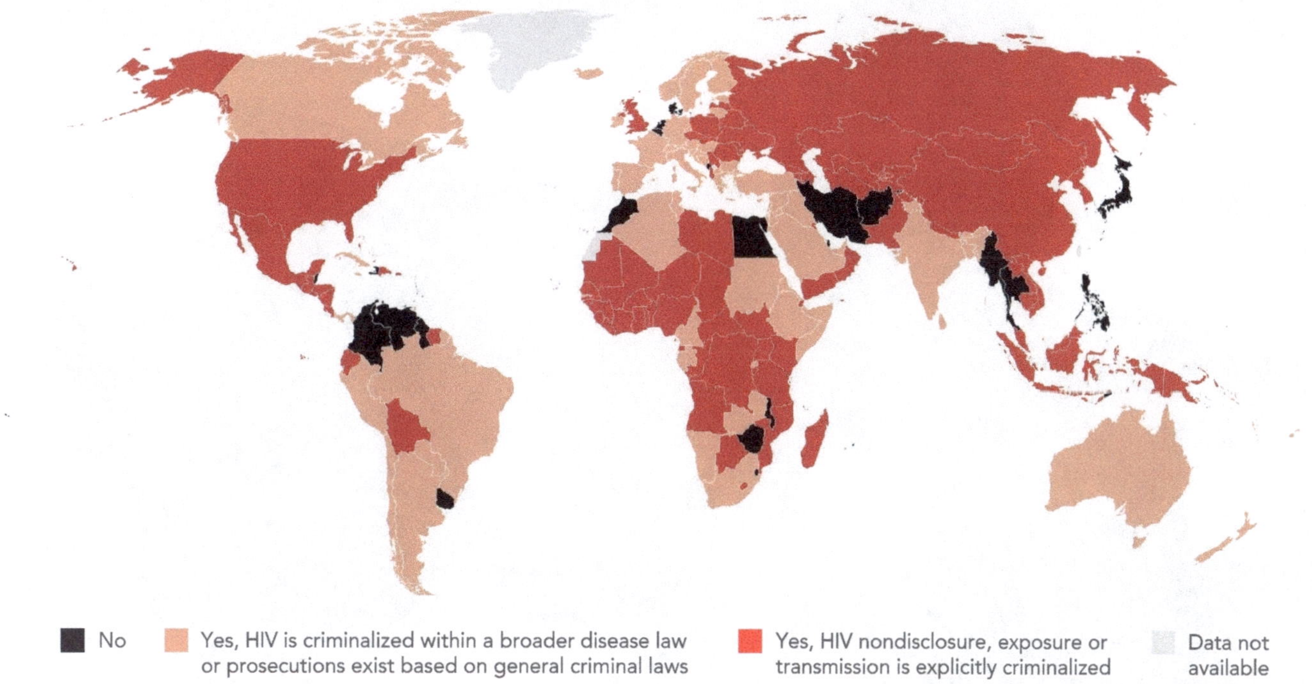

Source: National Commitments and Policy Instrument, 2017–2024 (http://lawsandpolicies.unaids.org/), supplemented by additional sources (see references in regional factsheets and http://lawsandpolicies.unaids.org/).

5 For real-time case tracking and law reform data, see the Global HIV Criminalisation Database (www.hivjustice.net).

The damage wrought to the HIV response by these punitive laws and policies is compounded by the declining space available for civil society to play its many invaluable roles. Burdens on civil society—including onerous registration procedures, restrictions on organizations receiving international assistance, and prohibitions of some civil society activities—are increasing worldwide, with CIVICUS (an international non-profit-making organization focused on civil rights and citizen action) reporting in 2024 that civil society was "under severe attack in 116 of 198 countries and territories" *(41)*.

International donors currently supply around 80% of funding for societal enablers, including human rights programmes addressing structural and systemic issues that increase HIV vulnerability and diminish access to HIV services. Further reductions in international HIV assistance have the potential to undermine efforts to promote, protect and fulfil the human rights of all people, and advance gender equality in the context of the HIV response with a direct impact on people's ability to access HIV and health services.

The vision of zero discrimination is anchored in the global 2025 targets, which include commitments to gender equality and the prevention of violence against women, girls and people from key populations. Yet, by 2024, the world was not on track to meet these targets *(42)*.

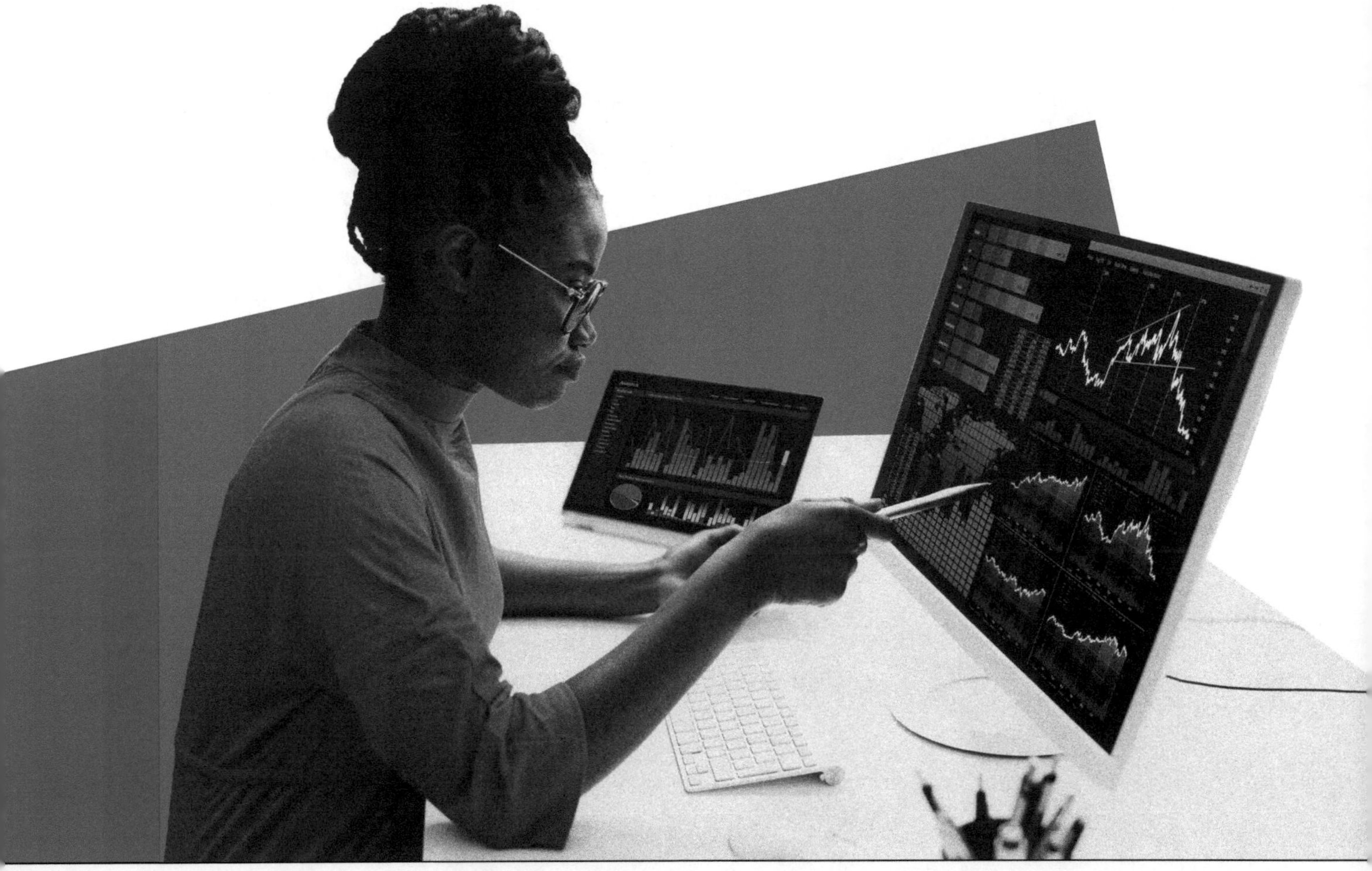

Key actions to break the inequality–pandemic cycle

Inequality and pandemics reinforce each other in a vicious cycle. High levels of inequality within and between countries are making the world more vulnerable to pandemics, making pandemics more economically disruptive and deadly, and making them last longer; pandemics in turn increase inequality *(43)*. This inequality–pandemic cycle is the key finding of two years of research by the Global Council on Inequality, AIDS and Pandemics.

Co-chaired by Nobel Laureate Joseph E Stiglitz, former First Lady of Namibia Monica Geingos and renowned epidemiologist Professor Sir Michael Marmot, the UNAIDS-convened Global Council has called for a new approach to health security capable of interrupting this cycle, which slows responses to the pandemics of today, including HIV, and undermines prevention and preparedness for future pandemics. The Global Council has recommended practical and achievable actions at the national and global levels that account for fundamental changes in the global order, including rapid declines in overseas development assistance. These recommendations include:

- immediate and comprehensive debt restructuring, starting with a pause until 2030 for countries in debt distress and facing pandemics including HIV—the freed-up fiscal space must be used to reduce inequalities, with investments in health and the social determinants of health, and not to bail out private creditors;
- surge social protection during health crises through a system ready to reach everyone, including people often excluded and made vulnerable, as one part of a multisectoral outbreak response capable of addressing social determinants;
- inspiring innovation with prizes instead of patents, and treating health innovations as global public goods in times of pandemics;
- making serious investments in the global south in research, development and manufacturing capacity to ensure all regions can produce health innovations quickly during global health emergencies;
- building greater trust, equality and efficiency in pandemic response by investing in community-led pandemic infrastructure in partnership with governments.

Factors limiting domestic fiscal space for HIV investments

Although no single set of actors can on its own ensure the long-term sustainability of the HIV response, securing and building on the gains made to date will require greater investment from domestic sources. Most low-income countries, however, especially those with heavy HIV burdens, lack the means to close HIV resource gaps. Fiscal space for increased domestic investments varies considerably among countries, with many countries confronting major barriers to mobilizing new financing for HIV programmes.

Heavy debt burdens undermine the capacity of many low- and middle-income countries to invest in HIV programmes. According to analyses by UNAIDS, most countries receiving external financing support are highly or very highly indebted. The ratio of debt to gross domestic product has increased in the post-COVID-19 period, with many countries now spending more on debt service than on health. In western and central Africa, for example, public debt service is on average 5.5 times greater than public health allocations, crowding out fiscal space for HIV investment (Figure 1.12).

Weaknesses and gaps in national systems for tax administration and collection diminish the capacity of countries to increase domestic investments in HIV. As a percentage of gross domestic product, African countries collect a lower share than countries that are members of the Organisation for Economic Co-operation and Development *(44)*.

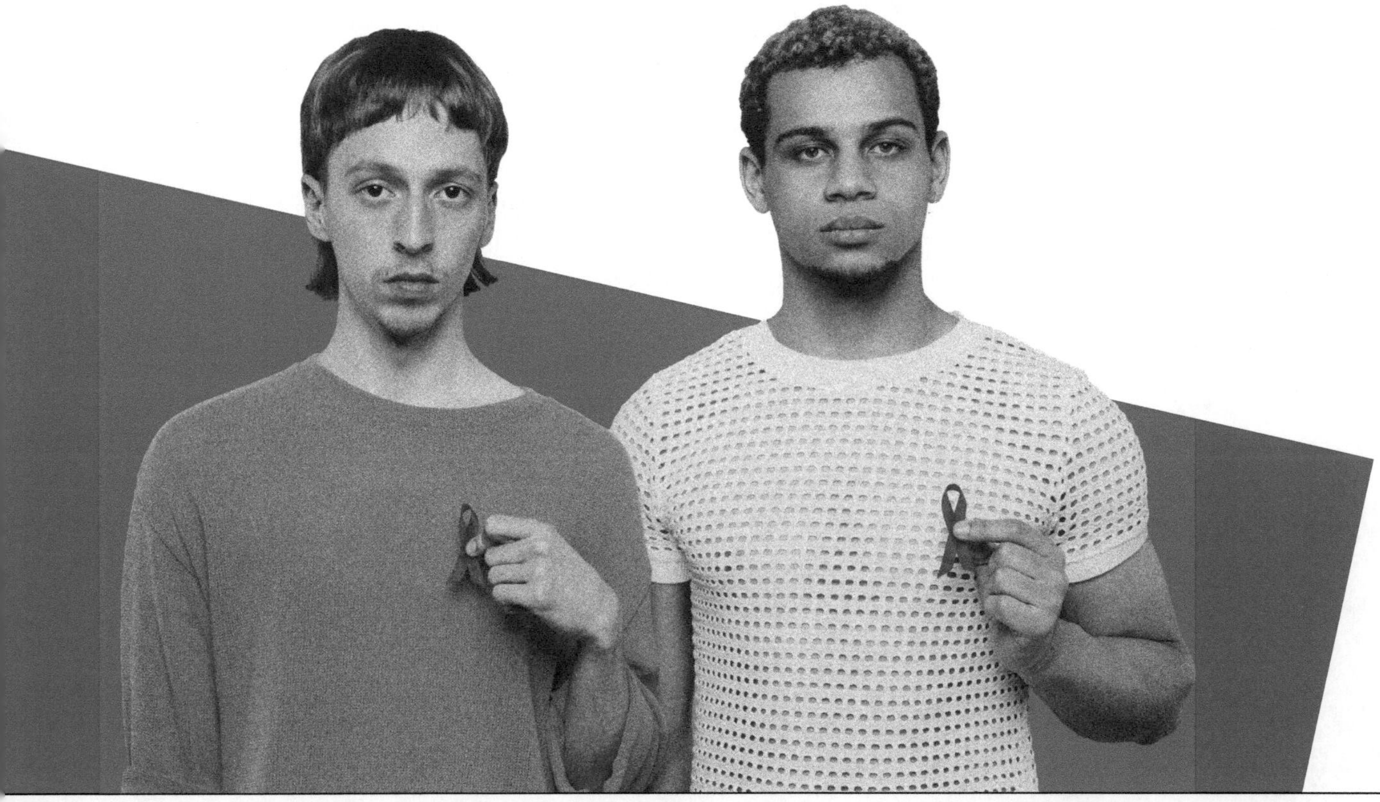

FIGURE 1.12

Dependency on external HIV funding in the context of high public debt servicing relative to health spending

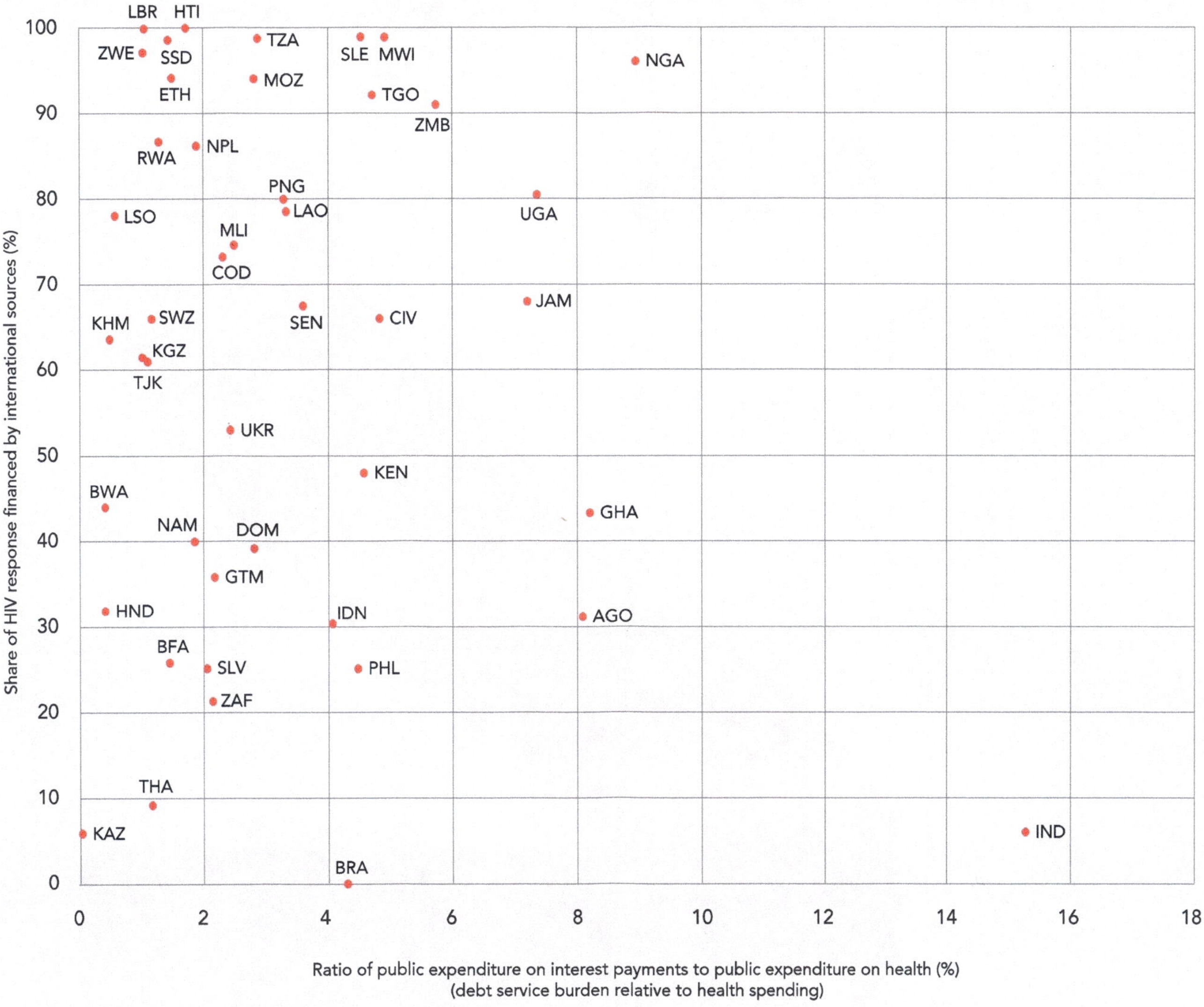

Note: Angola (AGO), Botswana (BWA), Brazil (BRA), Burkina Faso (BFA), Cambodia (KHM), Côte d'Ivoire (CIV), Democratic Republic of the Congo (COD), Dominican Republic (DOM), El Salvador (SLV), Ethiopia (ETH), Eswatini (SWZ), Ghana (GHA), Guatemala (GTM), Haiti (HTI), Honduras (HND), India (IND), Indonesia (IDN), Jamaica (JAM), Kazakhstan (KAZ), Kenya (KEN), Kyrgyzstan (KGZ), Lao People's Democratic Republic (LAO), Lesotho (LSO), Liberia (LBR), Malawi (MWI), Mali (MLI), Mozambique (MOZ), Namibia (NAM), Nepal (NPL), Nigeria (NGA), Papua New Guinea (PNG), Philippines (PHL), Rwanda (RWA), Senegal (SEN), Sierra Leone (SLE), South Africa (ZAF), South Sudan (SSD), Tajikistan (TJK), Thailand (THA), Togo (TGO), Uganda (UGA), Ukraine (UKR), United Republic of Tanzania (TZA), Zambia (ZMB), Zimbabwe (ZWE).
Source: Global AIDS Monitoring, UNAIDS-supported national AIDS spending assessments, 2019–2024.

Half of the countries assisted by external financing are experiencing fragility. Fiscal capacity to expand HIV funding is extremely limited under such circumstances because finite domestic resources are diverted to address immediate crises such as conflict, natural disasters and mass population displacement *(45)*.

Even in the best of circumstances, many low- and middle-income countries will struggle to allocate sufficient funding for HIV and other health services, in part due to the expanding array of national priorities requiring domestic investment. For example, adapting to the effects of climate change in low- and middle-income countries is projected to require total financing of US$ 387 billion per year this decade *(46)*.

2

Important signs of resilience in the HIV response

Although the impacts of funding cuts are severe, neither country governments nor communities have accepted these reductions passively. Instead, key actors at all levels are rapidly responding, developing and implementing measures to ensure the long-term sustainability of the response.

There is an emerging global consensus—supported by countries, donors, communities and other stakeholders—on the importance of transitioning national responses from donor dependence to greater sovereignty and national self-reliance. For the HIV response to be sustainable,[6] transformations need to take place to a degree unseen in the past two decades. These transformations have already started to take place, with shifts in systems, accelerated integration of the response into health and financial systems as they strengthen while incorporating community leadership and services, and growing domestic revenue mobilization and investments for health and HIV as international resources decline.

Regional action to ensure long-term sustainability

In 2025, African leaders, in the African Union Roadmap to 2030 and Beyond, pledged to ensure "diversified and sustainable financing" for HIV and other health programmes *(48)*. Also in 2025, in response to a sharp reduction in official development assistance, the African Union launched a new initiative to increase domestic health financing, with the aim of ensuring all countries across the region achieve the Abuja Declaration target of allocating at least 15% of government budgets to health. As of 2025, only three countries (Botswana, Cabo Verde, Rwanda) had consistently met the Abuja target *(49)*. The African Union acted in 2025 to create a new African Epidemic Fund to support countries in preparing for and responding to future health emergencies *(50)*.

Growing regional momentum for greater domestic health financing is building on a broader rethink of the global health and development paradigm. On the side of the United Nations General Assembly in September 2025, African leaders, convened by HE President Mahama of Ghana, launched the Accra Reset, calling for the creation of new governance and financing models for regional health and development. The Accra Reset acknowledges the need for continued health assistance but aims to "foster a new era of health sovereignty rooted in national ownership, investment and leadership" *(51)*. An extraordinary session of the African Union Assembly is being convened in December 2025 with the purpose

6 Sustainability is defined as a country's ability to have and use, in an enabling environment, person-centred, human rights-based and gender equality-based systems for health and equity, empowered and capable institutions and community-led organizations, and adequate, equitably distributed resources to reach and sustain the end of AIDS as a public health threat by 2030 and beyond, upholding the right to health for all *(47)*.

of securing a high-level declaration on the implementation of the African Union Roadmap to 2030 and Beyond: Sustaining the AIDS Response, ensuring systems strengthening and health security for the development of Africa *(52)*.

Regional leaders in Africa have embraced a framework for strengthening local manufacturing of medical products *(53)*. In October 2025, the Africa Center for Disease Control and Prevention launched an intelligence and analytic platform to bolster efforts to build greater pharmaceutical manufacturing capacity in the region *(54)*. The East Africa Community is in the process of implementing its second Regional Pharmaceutical Manufacturing Plan of Action *(55)*. Efforts to strengthen regional pharmaceutical manufacturing capacity are benefiting from an infusion of US$ 1.2 billion in support from the Global Alliance for Vaccines and Immunization (Gavi)-launched Africa Vaccine Manufacturing Accelerator initiative *(56)*. Strengthened manufacturing capacity in Africa is being buttressed by additional steps to maximize regional self-sufficiency with respect to HIV and other health commodities, including the launch in 2024 of the African Pooled Procurement Mechanism *(57)* and the creation in 2021 of the African Medicines Agency to enable validated medicines to reach people across the region as quickly as possible *(58)*.

Regional leadership to support long-term sustainability of the HIV response is evident outside of Africa as well. The Association of Southeast Asian Nations committed to "increase financing and adopt innovative financing mechanisms for the HIV response" *(59)*. In 2024, leaders in the Western Pacific Region developed an action framework to achieve universal health coverage, including through increased domestic public sector investments in health *(60)*. In 2025, leaders of the Caribbean Community reaffirmed the region's commitment to end AIDS as a public health threat, including through mobilization of increased resources *(61)*.

Swift action by countries to close funding gaps

Despite considerable limitations to fiscal space, many low- and middle-income countries have moved swiftly in 2025 to preserve HIV services and strengthen national responses. Although these increases in domestic investments do not fully compensate for reductions in international assistance, they have helped to mitigate some of the impacts of funding cuts. Twenty-six of 61 countries have reported plans to increase their domestic HIV budgets by 2026.[7]

In 2025, Nigeria approved marked increases in its health budget and spending on HIV treatment programmes *(62)*. Uganda has taken steps to double its domestic spending on health *(63)*. Côte d'Ivoire has committed to increase

7 Twenty-six of the 61 countries reporting to UNAIDS on forecasted budget trends for 2026 have stated they expect to increase their domestic public HIV budgets: Bhutan, Bolivia (Plurinational State of), Brazil, Dominican Republic, Namibia, Pakistan, Republic of Moldova, Tajikistan, Timor-Leste (<5% increase); Algeria, Azerbaijan, Belarus, Central African Republic, Cuba, Egypt, Georgia, Kazakhstan, Kenya, Nigeria, Thailand, United Republic of Tanzania (5–10% increase); Democratic Republic of the Congo, Ethiopia, Mali, Niger (>10% increase), Uganda.

its domestic investments in HIV services in 2025 (by US$ 60 million to US$ 65 million) and in 2026 and beyond (by US$ 80 million to US$ 85 million annually) *(64)*. South Africa has increased its domestic HIV investments by US$ 33 million to help mitigate the effects of reduced donor support *(65)*. The United Republic of Tanzania is dedicating increases in various excise taxes to reduce the impact of HIV funding cuts *(66)*. A review of domestic resource mobilization strategies in seven African countries (Ethiopia, Kenya, Malawi, Nigeria, United Republic of Tanzania, Zambia, Zimbabwe) found that countries are pursuing a range of strategies to mitigate the effects of potential reductions in donor support, including increased domestic financing, concessional loans, public–private partnerships and earmarked taxes *(67)*.

Leadership to minimize the effects of funding shortfalls on HIV services is visible in other regions as well. The Government of Guatemala has stepped in after donor support declined to ensure continuity of HIV services *(68)*. Viet Nam has committed to prioritize domestic resources, including its national health insurance scheme, to minimize disruptions of funding cuts to the national response *(69)*.

In a number of countries, strong national leadership on HIV funding has helped to mitigate the impact of donor cuts on HIV services (see Figure 1.9). Kenya, which has steadily increased its domestic investments in HIV services in recent years *(70)*, has succeeded in minimizing the effects of donor cuts on uptake of antiretroviral therapy and HIV testing services, although the number of people receiving PrEP in Kenya declined during the first six months of 2025. There is also evidence that the impacts of reductions in donor support on access to HIV services have been somewhat less pronounced in countries where antiretroviral therapy had already been integrated into national health insurance schemes, such as the Philippines, Thailand and Viet Nam.

In 2024, before the funding cuts of 2025, UNAIDS and partners began developing a new approach to sustainability planning for the HIV response. This approach, reflected in the development of national HIV response sustainability roadmaps, relies on inclusive, participatory "country driven and owned processes [to] drive sustainable HIV response transformations" *(71)*.

More than 30 countries, with support from UNAIDS and partners, are developing clear, actionable roadmaps to end AIDS as a public health threat and to secure HIV-related gains across future years. All sustainability roadmaps created to date include strong commitments to increase domestic financing for HIV programmes. Uganda, for example, pledges to increase the share of HIV spending financed through domestic resources from 20% currently to 50% by 2040 *(72)*. Togo's roadmap sets the goal to increase domestic financing of the HIV response from 15% to 50% by 2030 *(73)*. From the current low level of 2% domestic financing of HIV response activities, Malawi has established the goal of increasing the domestic share to 30–50% by 2030 *(74)*. Zambia calls for the introduction of legislation to establish a health fund that includes HIV services in its public health package *(75)*. Lesotho has established a target of ensuring domestic financing of at least 90% of HIV commodities and laboratory reagents (from 30% currently), including through the creation of a national HIV and tuberculosis (TB) fund *(76)*. Ghana proposes that the levy created for COVID-19 be transformed into a sustainable pandemic levy fund, with an earmarked allocation for HIV response activities *(77)*.

Using the Rapid AIDS Response Tool (RAFT) to respond to the crisis

With UNAIDS support, countries are developing strategies to manage the sudden funding losses.

Thirty-two countries, two regional programmes, Global Fund teams and partners used the UNAIDS Rapid AIDS Financing Tool (RAFT) to guide emergency resource mobilization, reprogramming and budget integration by:

- analysing the impact of the funding freeze impacts on HIV spending, programmes, procurement, human resources and services;
- prioritizing and costing interventions using local data (e.g. health worker salary scales), and estimating the funding gap.

Malawi used RAFT to inform the additional allocation of US$ 11 million to the Ministry of Health in the 2025 budget to recruit 6000 staff currently covered by donor-funded programmes onto the government payroll. El Salvador used RAFT to prioritize 28% of the PEPFAR 2024–2025 budget for immediate transition action, ensuring the sustainability of essential health-care workers who provide HIV care and treatment services. Zimbabwe also leveraged RAFT to assess the impact of the funding freeze, identify critical policy shifts, and prioritize and advocate for domestic investments to offset donor funding reductions. In addition to catalysing mobilization of new domestic funding, RAFT also enables countries to identify strategies for simplifying service delivery and optimizing service outcomes, including through effective scale-up of advances in HIV prevention and treatment technologies, such as long-acting injectable regimens.

For more information, see https://sustainability.unaids.org

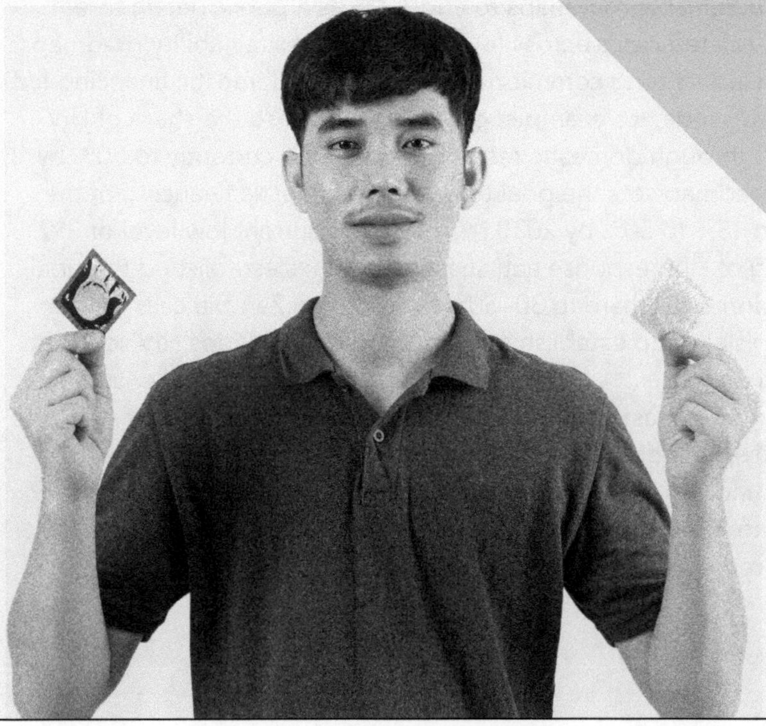

Innovative high-level leadership to strengthen and sustain the HIV response in Uganda

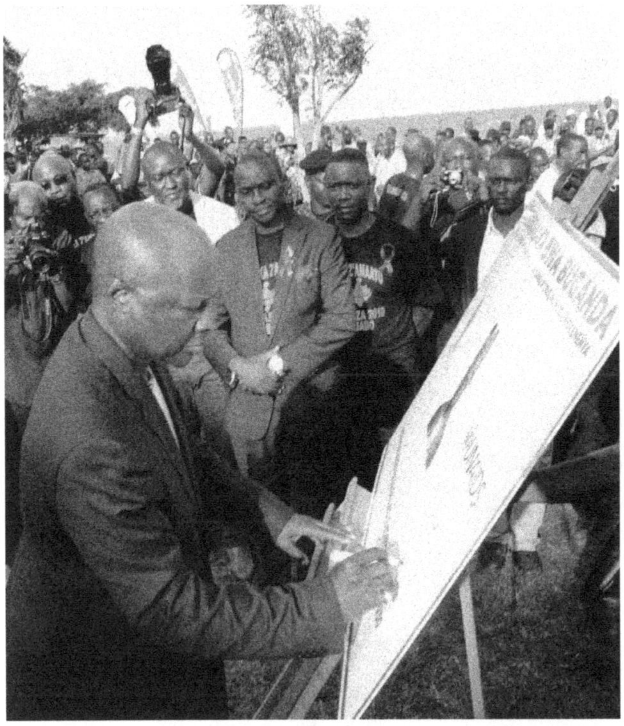

In the traditional kingdom of the Buganda people within present-day Uganda, the King, His Majesty Mutebi II, has championed health and well-being over the course of his reign, including through a series of multicomponent campaigns that aim to instil healthy social norms and health-seeking behaviours. In 2017, UNAIDS appointed the King as a UNAIDS Goodwill Ambassador on ending AIDS in eastern and southern Africa.

The King's HIV advocacy campaign, Abaami Munyenye ("Men are Stars"), has focused on men and boys aged 15–49 years who live in districts with a high HIV burden. The campaign piggybacked major sporting events, including a marathon to celebrate the King's birthday, which attracted 50 000–60 000 participants (85% male), and the Malaza football cup, which attracted 20 000–30 000 fans. The fees paid by participants at these events raised funds to support the health services promoted for men and boys.

The campaign has had a clear positive impact on HIV outcomes in Buganda. From 2016 to 2020, the percentage of people living with HIV who knew their HIV status rose from 89% to 94%, HIV treatment coverage increased from 64% to 92%, and the number of new HIV infections declined by 52%.

As the King's previous health promotion campaigns had been time-limited (typically running for three years), there was consideration in 2025 of creating a new campaign to replace the HIV campaign. With donor cutbacks potentially jeopardizing national momentum towards HIV epidemic control, however, the King determined that now was not the time to move on from the HIV response. As a result, the campaign to improve HIV outcomes is now continuing across the kingdom through 2030.

Multisectoral resilience to funding cuts in Guatemala

In 2025, cuts in international support for the HIV response in Guatemala and a reduced HIV allocation from the Global Fund caused immediate challenges for the HIV response because a substantial portion of the personnel at HIV comprehensive care units and community outreach workers that help facilitate and maintain access to services for people from key populations have long been funded by external donors. Some services were curtailed or discontinued altogether in clinics affected by the cuts, and remaining service providers struggled to absorb clients who had lost their service access.

In response to these cuts in external funding, the Ministry of Health stepped in to ensure continuity of care by covering the salaries of 81 members of staff, thereby sustaining the operation of numerous HIV comprehensive care units and guaranteeing service delivery to thousands of people nationwide. When a key implementer and PrEP provider lost its financing, the Government intervened to fill the gap. Gaps persist, however, with respect to prevention programmes for people from key populations.

Community-led responses have also stepped into the breach created by the loss of international assistance. Colectivo Amigos contra el Sida (CAS), an organization focused on HIV prevention among gay men and other men who have sex with men and transgender women, moved to assume responsibility for supporting PrEP delivery to clients of a large PrEP programme that lost its funding. CAS collects voluntary donations for services from clients who can afford to pay, which helps to co-finance operational costs that are no longer covered by international donors.

Planning for sustainability is an urgent priority for Guatemala. The Global Fund is set to phase out its support given Guatemala's status as an upper-middle-income country. Furthermore, UNAIDS has collaborated with the Ministry of Health and the national AIDS programme to roll out the UNAIDS Rapid AIDS Financing Tool, aimed at facilitating decision-making and actions in response to cuts in United States cooperation.

Recognizing the essential role played by community-led responses, UNAIDS is collaborating with the Global Fund to help build the knowledge and capacity of civil society organizations to lobby more effectively for greater domestic resources.

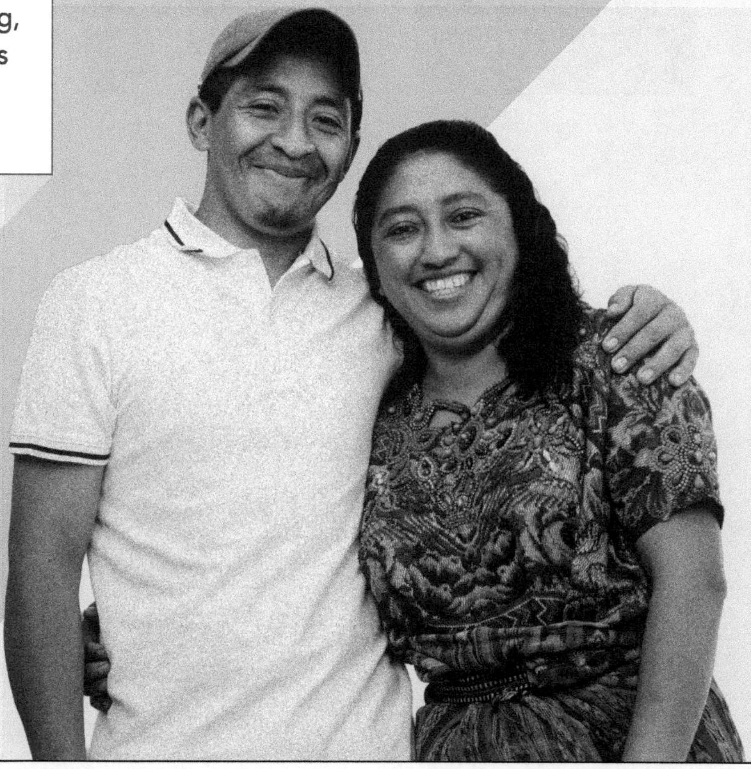

Collective action to integrate, strengthen and sustain the national HIV response in Nigeria

Nigeria has made important strides towards ending its national HIV epidemic. In 2024, the country was within reach of the 95–95–95 targets, and the annual number of new HIV infections was 67% lower than in 2010. Nigeria's progress came under serious threat in 2025 following the pause in PEPFAR funding and the dismantlement of USAID. Nigeria has long relied on external partners for more than 80% of the costs of its national HIV response *(78)*.

In the face of funding uncertainties, the federal Government of Nigeria stepped up decisively to allocate an additional US$ 200 million in domestic funding to safeguard and sustain HIV treatment services. "President Bola Ahmed Tinubu is committed to transforming the sector by strengthening national systems, securing local financing, and exploring other funding sources to ensure that patients do not lose access to their treatment," stated Dr Muhammad Ali Pate, Coordinating Minister of Health and Social Welfare *(79)*.

Before the funding disruptions in January and February 2025, the Government had also begun working with communities and other stakeholders to lay the foundation for long-term sustainability of the HIV response, explains Dr Temitope Ilori, Director General of the National Agency for the Control of AIDS. Through an inclusive, data-driven process, Nigeria has articulated a roadmap to ensure the sustainability of the national response to HIV.

"We are working towards sustainability, but we are not there yet," says Dr Ilori. "We still need that partnership, that collaboration [with United States and other external donors]."

Work is also under way to promote domestic production of HIV commodities, including recently signed memoranda of understanding with the private sector for the local production of HIV test kits and antiretroviral medicines.

Although national leadership has helped to mitigate some of the effects of the loss of donor support, governmental and nongovernmental informants note the continuing negative effects of funding cuts on HIV responses for people from key populations. Aniedi Akplan, Chair of the Drug Harm Reduction Advocacy Network, reports that a planned expansion of harm reduction programmes has been scrapped due to the loss of funding, with such services now limited to only four Nigerian states.

Although national leadership has helped preserve HIV treatment services, HIV prevention services have been much more heavily affected. "There are not many HIV prevention activities happening across the country now, especially for key populations," says Abdulkadir Ibrahim, national coordinator of the Network of People Living with HIV/AIDS in Nigeria.

Community resilience

Around the world, community-led responses are reeling from the loss of essential funding, most of which has long been provided by external donors. But there are also encouraging signs of resilience from community-led partners.

In Zimbabwe, the community-led GALZ has worked to preserve and improve the access of LGBTQI+ people to health care in Harare, Masvingo and Mutare by strengthening collaboration with the national health ministry and with municipal governments *(80)*. In Uganda, when funding cuts forced the closure of offices of the national network of people living with HIV, the Uganda AIDS Commission stepped in to provide office space and ensure continuation of the network (personal communication, FR Anam, Global Network of People Living with HIV, 27 October 2025). NEPHAK, a national network of people living with or at risk of HIV in Kenya, is actively advocating for integration of HIV into general medical care and to include HIV treatment in the package of services covered by the national health insurance programme *(81)*.

When the funding cuts resulted in the loss of 60–70% of HIV service funding for the Centre for Sexual Health, HIV and AIDS Research, a leading provider of PrEP, the organization moved quickly to obtain funding from the Gates Foundation and ViiV to mitigate the effects of funding reductions (personal communication, B Chingombe, CESHAAR Zimbabwe, 7 November 2025). In Viet Nam, the key population-led Lighthouse has piloted tiered co-payment models for PrEP to mitigate the effects of donor cuts and also provided financial support to community members negatively affected by service cutbacks (personal communication, T Doan, Lighthouse, Viet Nam, 27 October 2025). The global HIV response stands at a crossroads. "Across the Frontline AIDS partnership, 1.6 million people lost access to HIV prevention and treatment this year, and 27 organizations were forced to shut lifesaving HIV services," says Leora Pillay of Frontine AIDS, 20 November 2025. "In the wake of the funding crisis, we've launched our Transition Initiative, bringing community-led and civil society partners together to push for national HIV responses which are strong, sustainably financed, and include the people and communities at highest risk of HIV," she says.

These examples of community resilience, although inspiring, cannot obscure the harsh climates in which community-led responses are working, with funding rapidly disappearing and punitive policies proliferating. Almost by definition, communities affected by HIV lack the financial resources available to national governments, donor agencies and large implementing partners. Relying on unpaid volunteer efforts by communities is neither just nor sustainable.

All country roadmaps for HIV response sustainability that have been developed to date prioritize increasing financial support for community-led interventions and organizations, with nearly all calling for action to establish robust mechanisms for social contracting. Uganda, for example, aims to establish social contracting of civil society organizations by 2025 and ensure at least 25% of civil society organizations providing services in high-burden districts receive domestic financing by 2040 *(72)*. Some country roadmaps aim to relax regulatory restrictions that prevent community-led organizations from registering and receiving funding, and all roadmaps emphasize strengthening community-led monitoring as a basis for accountability and for enhancing HIV and other health services.

Challenges and resilience among networks of people living with HIV

At the global, regional and country levels, networks of people living with HIV have fulfilled an essential role in the HIV response. These networks not only offer social, emotional and practical support for people living with HIV, but also contribute to the development, implementation and monitoring of national HIV responses.

Declining donor support has had major negative effects on networks of people living with HIV, including substantial reductions in staffing. According to Florence Riako Anam, Co-executive Director of the Global Network of People Living with HIV (GNP+), national networks have lost staff and peer educators in countries including Indonesia, Nigeria, Rwanda, Uganda and Zimbabwe, and some networks have been forced to close their doors.

Recognizing the threat posed to critical HIV support and advocacy networks, 80 people living with HIV from 18 countries and six regions convened in Nairobi in April 2025 for the People Living with HIV leadership summit sponsored by GNP+. With the aim of assessing the state of leadership among people living with HIV and charting a pathway towards sustainability of the HIV response, the summit embraced a set of solidarity principles. Calling for a reimagining of advocacy by people living with HIV, the leaders proposed to "move from antagonistic to collaborative engagement with national governments, all partners and decision-makers".

"What we saw beginning in January [2025—when PEPFAR funding was interrupted] was that networks of people living with HIV have been engaging with governments to respond and adapt changes to HIV services, a unique opportunity for securing responsive services for people living with HIV and those affected," Riako Anam says. "Networks have built technical capacity and relationships over time ... and now we need to step up and make sure that systems are adapted to our needs. We can critique these systems later, but now we have to contextually build them together with national governments."

Integrating HIV services to improve outcomes and buttress long-term sustainability

The HIV response has been a global pioneer in integrated, person-centred health service models *(82)*. Integrating HIV services with non-HIV-specific health services has been found to improve health outcomes and make health systems more effective *(83)*. Among the 152 countries with available data, about a quarter have integrated their HIV responses with broader health strategies. Integration at the point of care can make it easier and less costly for people to access multiple health services. Integration is also expected to generate savings for service providers, if more versatile service platforms increase coverage and reduce costs. Integration of systems (e.g. supply chains, laboratories, human resources, information systems, financing channels, programme management) has the potential to boost efficiencies, generate cost savings, and improve the overall functioning of health systems.

There is good evidence supporting many of these expectations. A meta-analysis of 114 studies, mostly in sub-Saharan Africa, reported that both HIV and other health outcomes were better in integrated services than in separated services and the uptake of non-HIV services tended to rise. Country studies report increased rates of HIV testing *(83)* and high acceptability of cervical cancer screening *(84)*, Improvements in the linked delivery of HIV and TB services have led to a decline in the number of TB-related deaths, down by 76% between 2010 and 2024 *(85)*.

The steadily rising median age of people living with HIV is providing additional impetus for HIV service integration because people living with HIV are increasingly vulnerable over time to noncommunicable diseases *(86, 87)*. In 2025, the World Health Organization (WHO) updated its guidelines on HIV service delivery to encourage greater integration of HIV with services for diabetes, hypertension and mental health and to strengthen person-centred service delivery that streamlines delivery and ensures care is responsive to clients' preferences and circumstances *(88)*.

Countries are moving to carry the HIV service integration agenda even further. For the national sustainability roadmaps developed thus far, transitioning HIV-related services and systems to national ownership, oversight and financing is a central aim. For example, the sustainability roadmap of the United Republic of Tanzania pledges to transition from a "national to a community-based and community-led people-centred response" *(89)*, and Namibia commits to expanding primary health care and person-centred delivery models, with a focus on rural and community levels in a large, sparsely populated country *(90)*.

Country roadmaps emphasize the importance of pursuing service integration in a careful, rights-based, deliberative manner *(91)*. As part of a robust person-centred health system, national roadmaps also pledge to ensure strong national data systems.

In the context of rapidly integrating responses, it is important to ensure integrated services preserve person-centred approaches and protect human rights and gender equality. These approaches are critical to sustain the demand and coverage of services. This is particularly important for people from key populations and for people living with HIV (especially women), who are exposed to heightened stigma and discrimination when seeking health services *(92)*. A December 2025 report from Mozambique states that sex workers, gay men and other men who have sex with men, trans and gender diverse people and people who use drugs now face stigma and discrimination in overburdened public clinics. People from criminalized populations have reported being judged and humiliated, which has eroded trust and discouraged them from returning to these clinics *(5)*. A balance must be struck between greater integration and preserving the community-driven accountability and engagement that make HIV programmes successful, including community-led monitoring, community-led research and advocacy, community engagement in decision-making and community-led service delivery *(92)*.

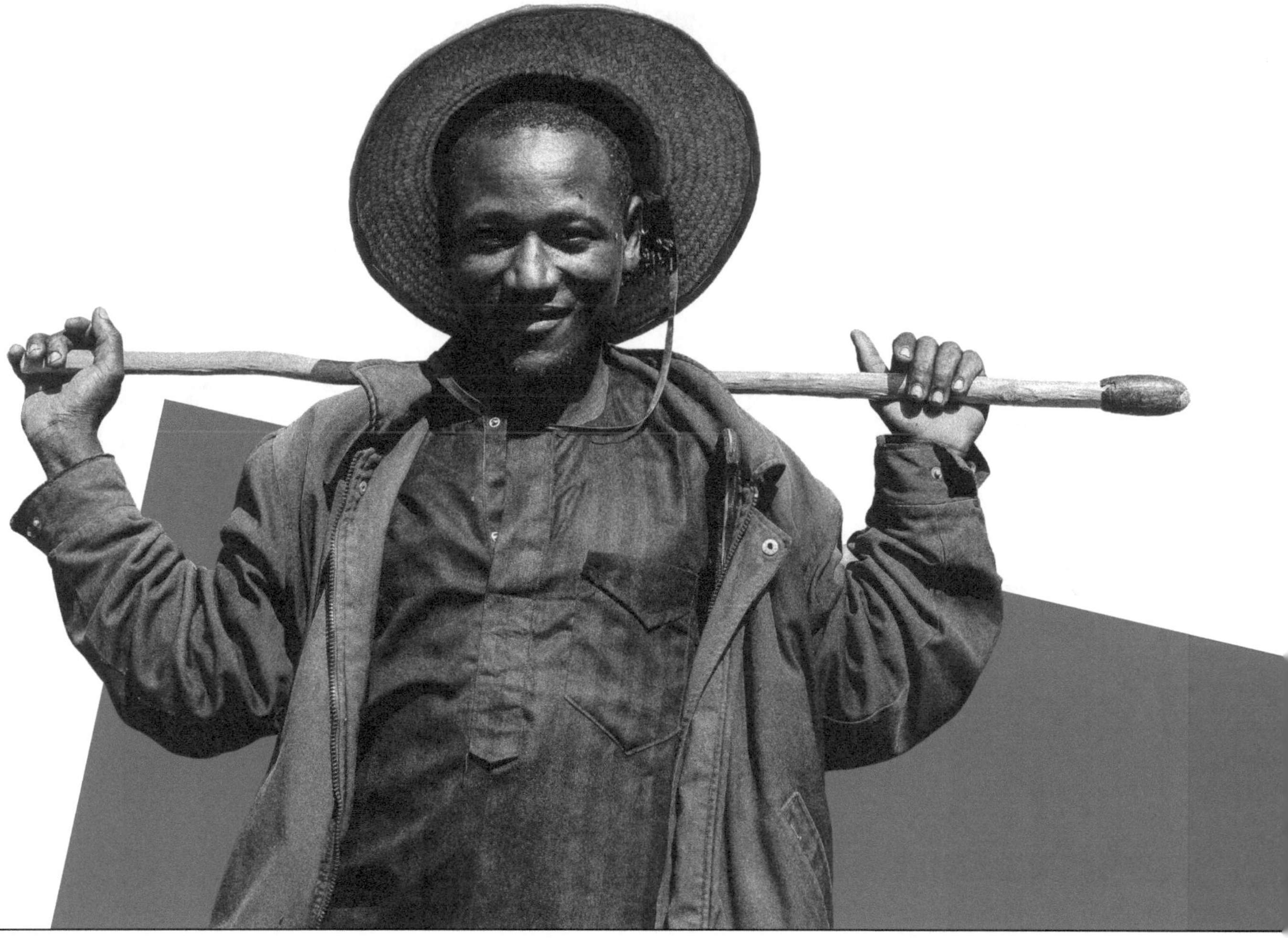

3

Towards a sustainable HIV response: reaffirming global solidarity

Shared responsibility and global solidarity have been the foundations on which the global HIV response has achieved its historic reductions in numbers of new HIV infections and AIDS-related deaths. As we transition to a new era of solidarity, shared responsibility and global solidarity will remain essential to hopes for ending AIDS. Unless the world pulls together to overcome the growing financing, human rights and programmatic challenges confronting the HIV response, we will miss the opportunity to end AIDS as a public health threat.

The UNAIDS Joint Programme urges the global community to take immediate and decisive action to close HIV-related resource gaps. This will require collaboration and action by a broad array of stakeholders—at the global, regional and national levels—and openness to new, innovative approaches to mobilize new funding and optimize impact by enhancing the efficient use of available resources.

Bringing essential HIV programmes to the people who need them

Using the powerfully effective prevention and treatment tools that are available is essential to reduce the number of new HIV infections to as low a level as possible. Sharply lowering HIV incidence saves lives and reduces future financial outlays for HIV treatment and care and enables a careful focusing of surveillance and prevention efforts on people with the greatest vulnerability to HIV acquisition.

Maximizing HIV viral suppression through timely HIV diagnosis, linkage to care and strong treatment adherence are cornerstones of hopes to end AIDS as a public health threat. According to a 10-year longitudinal study among gay men and other men who have sex with men in Australia, every 1% increase in population prevalence of HIV viral suppression resulted in a 6% decrease in HIV incidence *(93)*.

New mathematical modelling commissioned by UNAIDS underscores the critical importance of further programmatic scale-up and maintenance of very high service coverage levels. This modelling, however, also demonstrates that HIV treatment, although essential, will not on its own end AIDS. Scaled-up HIV treatment must be complemented by an equally robust commitment to bring HIV prevention services to everyone who needs them.

Donor cuts in 2025, combined with the early responses of countries to these reductions, may mean testing and treatment programmes struggle to build on their 2024 coverage levels, and access to HIV prevention services has already declined markedly. Modelling the impact of these funding cuts, UNAIDS projects that in 2030 there would be 1.4 million annual new HIV infections. Over the period 2025–2030 this would result in an additional 3.9 million people newly acquiring HIV, compared with a scenario of reaching the global HIV targets by 2030 (Figure 3.1). This demonstrates the importance of further HIV service scale-up and the urgent need to bring prevention coverage up to the much higher levels reported for HIV testing and treatment.

FIGURE 3.1

Number of people acquiring HIV, 2020–2024, and projected scenarios, 2025–2030, global.

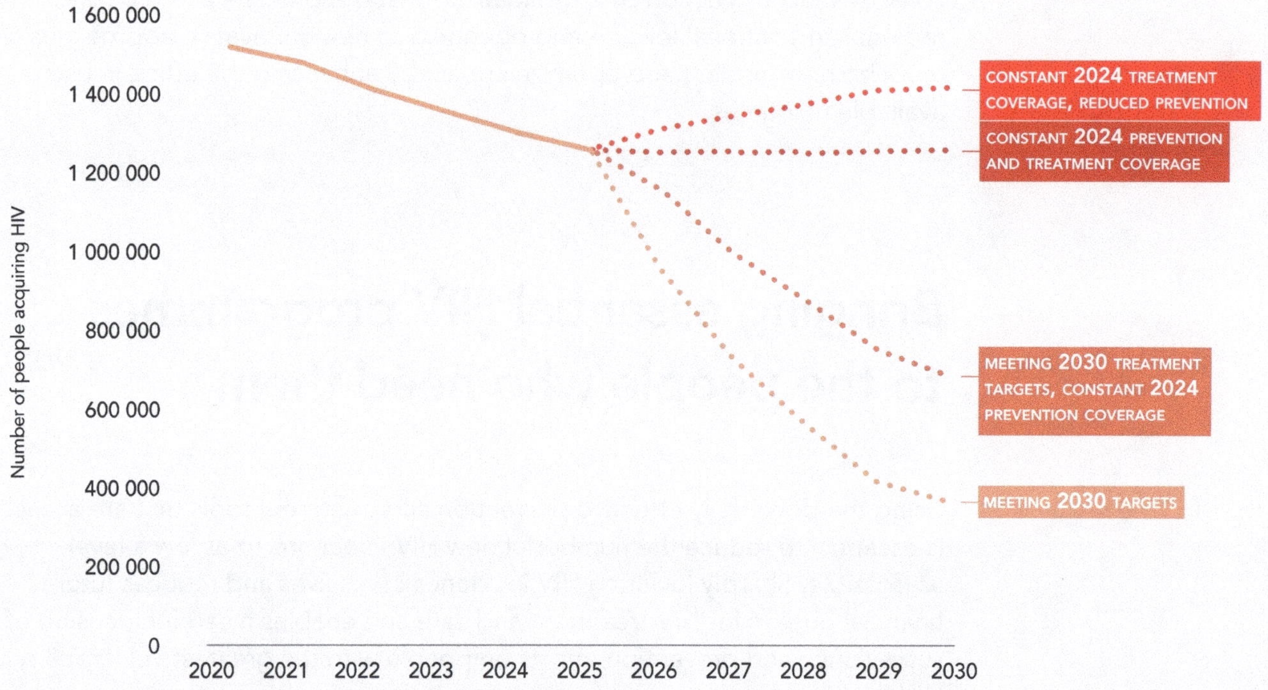

Source: 2025 UNAIDS epidemiological estimates and Goals projections.

Reduced global funding for the HIV response is likely to increase the number of new HIV infections and undermine efforts to end AIDS as a public health threat, essentially returning the global epidemic to its 2020, state erasing years of public health gains.

A new global AIDS strategy: a blueprint to leverage powerful tools to end AIDS

The Global AIDS Strategy 2026–2031, to be adopted by the UNAIDS Programme Coordinating Board in December 2025 and endorsed by United Nations Member States at the United Nations General Assembly high-level meeting on HIV and AIDS in June 2026, aims to catalyse a renewed commitment to end AIDS as a public health threat by 2030 and sustain gains beyond 2030. The new Strategy will accomplish this by combining country leadership of inclusive national responses, progress in reducing inequalities, upholding rights of all people in the context of HIV, and elevating community leadership across all levels and aspects of the response. To forge consensus on the new Strategy, UNAIDS convened a broad range of strategy consultations with diverse stakeholders, including thousands of government officials, communities, the private sector and research organizations.

The new Strategy is person-centred and has fewer focused targets. It emphasizes transitioning from vertical HIV programmes to HIV service integration in national programmes and further expanding the range of service approaches to meet people's needs, including self-care, community-led programmes, promotion of human rights, gender equality, enabling environments and differentiated service delivery (Figure 3.2).

FIGURE 3.2

2026–2031 Global AIDS Strategy

THE STRATEGY IS STRUCTURED AROUND THREE PRIORITIES AND EIGHT RESULT AREAS

Three priorities and eight results areas are recommended to build a sustainable response and end AIDS as a public health threat by 2030

PRIORITY 1
SUSTAIN THE RESPONSE

Country-led, resilient and ready for the future

- **RESULT AREA 1:** Ensure financing for people-centred global and national HIV responses
- **RESULT AREA 2:** Integrate HIV interventions and HIV-related health and community systems with primary health care, broader health systems and key non-health sectors
- **RESULT AREA 3:** Invest in essential information systems and data collection in multiple sectors, including communities

PRIORITY 2
PEOPLE-FOCUSED SERVICES

Equity, dignity and access

- **RESULT AREA 4:** Scale up HIV prevention options that bring together biomedical, structural, community and behavioural interventions
- **RESULT AREA 5:** Guarantee equitable access to available, accessible, acceptable and high-quality HIV testing, treatment and care
- **RESULT AREA 6:** End stigma and discrimination and uphold human rights and gender equality in the HIV response
- **RESULT AREA 7:** Ensure equitable access to scientific, medical and technological innovations in HIV prevention, testing, treatment and care

PRIORITY 3
COMMUNITY LEADERSHIP

Empowered communities leading the HIV response

- **RESULT AREA 8:** Empower communities to lead

LOCAL, REGIONAL AND MULTILATERAL ACTION TO END AIDS

Scaling up HIV prevention efforts is of overriding importance in all regions—but especially in settings where numbers of new HIV infections are on the rise. Across sub-Saharan Africa, adolescent girls and young women remain at exceptionally high risk of acquiring HIV, underscoring the need for focused efforts and approaches to address the many needs of this diverse population. The rising proportion of new HIV infections among people from key populations and their partners (see Chapter 1) highlights the need to improve HIV prevention, testing, treatment and care for all.

Resource mobilization is a priority in all settings, but the strategies different countries may want to use to ensure financing for person-centred HIV responses will vary, taking into account factors such as national economic conditions and debt burden.

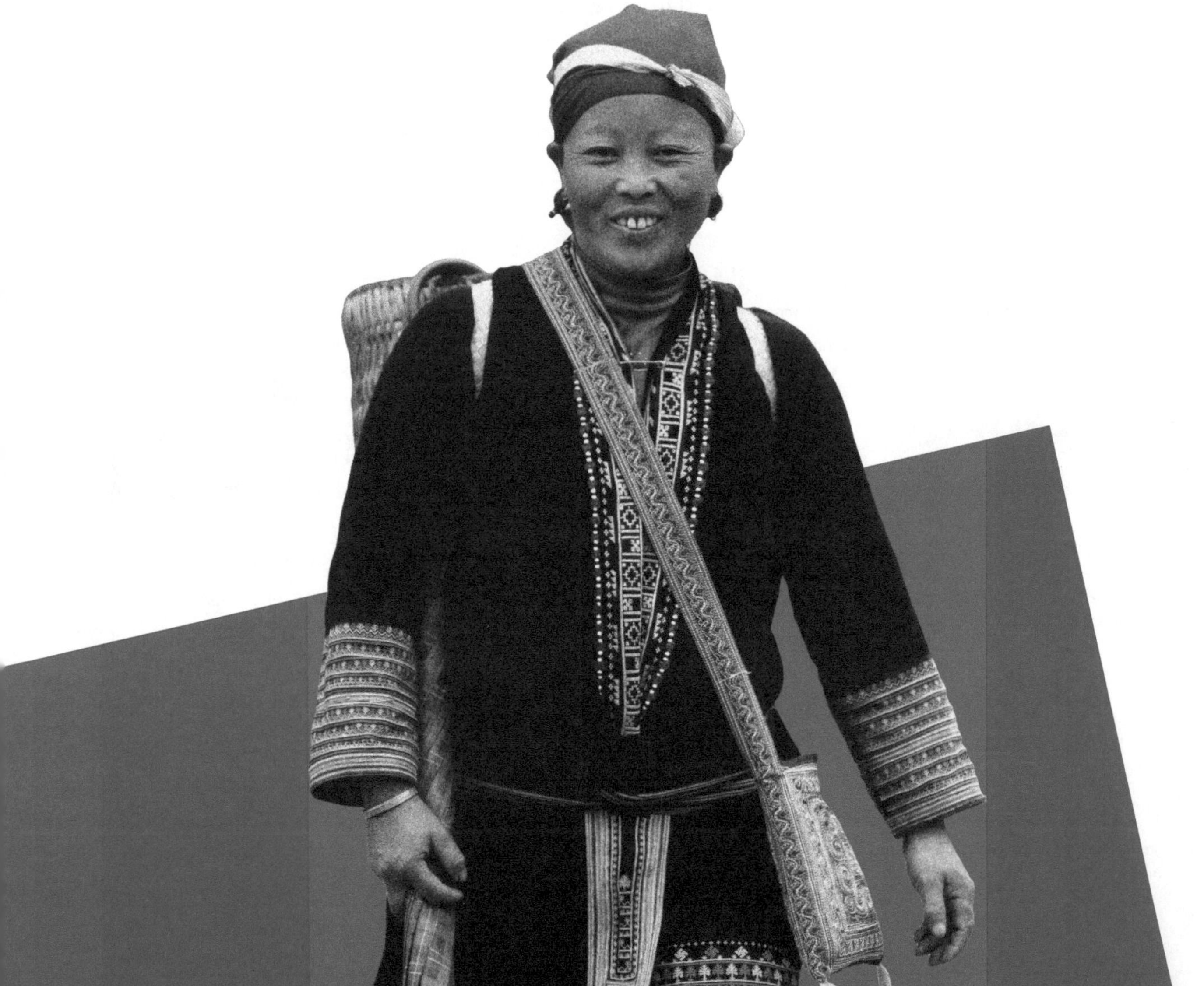

IMPLEMENTING THE GLOBAL AIDS STRATEGY 2026–2031: WHAT CAN BE ACHIEVED

The Global AIDS Strategy 2026–2031 includes 16 top-line targets to be achieved by 2030 (Figure 3.3). An additional 50 second-tier targets have been developed for the key outcomes needed to achieve the 16 top-line targets.

FIGURE 3.3

The 16 topline targets to end AIDS as a public health threat by 2030 and ensure sustainability of the HIV response post-2030[a]

Ensure available, accessible, acceptable and high-quality HIV treatment and care for people living with HIV	• 95% of people living with HIV know their HIV status • 95% of people living with HIV who know their HIV status receive treatment • 95% of people living with HIV who are on treatment have a suppressed viral load
Scale up HIV prevention options that bring together biomedical, structural and behavioural interventions	• 90% of people in need of prevention use prevention options (PrEP, PEP, condoms, needle–syringe programmes, opioid agonist maintenance therapy)
End stigma and discrimination and uphold human rights and gender equality in the HIV response	• <10% of people living with HIV and people from key and vulnerable populations experience stigma and discrimination • <10% experience gender inequality or violence • <10% of countries have punitive legal and policy environments that restrict access to services
Ensure community leadership in the HIV response	• Community led-organizations deliver 30% of testing and treatment support services • Community led-organizations deliver 80% of prevention options • Community led-organizations deliver 60% of societal enabler programmes
Integrate HIV services, with primary health care, broader health systems and other sectors	• 95% of people receiving HIV prevention or treatment services also receive needed sexual and reproductive health services (including for sexually transmitted infections) • 95% of pregnant women living with HIV and their newborns receive maternal and newborn care that integrates or links to comprehensive HIV services, including for prevention of HIV and hepatitis B virus and treatment of syphilis
Ensure sustainable financing for person-centred national and global HIV responses	• Reduce out-of-pocket expenses for HIV in line with universal health coverage • Increase percentage of HIV expenditure that is domestic • US$21.9 billion mobilized for HIV investments for low- and middle-income countries • All countries have access to equitable pricing for diagnostics and therapeutics

By 2030, reduce new HIV infections by 90% from 2010 and continued 5% decline per year after 2030

Reduce AIDS-related deaths by 90% from 2010

Ensure sustainability of the HIV response after 2030

PEP: post-exposure prophylaxis; **PrEP:** pre-exposure prophylaxis.

a The targets will be disaggregated as appropriate by gender, age and key population.

FUNDING REQUIRED TO ACHIEVE THE 2030 TARGETS

UNAIDS estimates that US$ 21.9 billion will be needed annually through 2030 to achieve the global HIV targets in low- and middle-income countries (Figure 3.4). The annual price tag for a sound, effective global response has fallen by $7.4 billion (from US$29.3 billion in 2021) due to several positive factors, including reductions in prices of antiretroviral medicines, validation and scale-up of simplified treatment regimens and service delivery models, improved approaches to effectively target interventions based on HIV risk, and graduation of a number of countries to high-income status (not costed here).

Resource needs for achieving the 2030 targets differ among countries and regions, with upper-middle-income countries accounting for 46% of projected resources needs in 2026–2030, followed by lower-middle-income countries (34%) and low-income countries (20%). HIV resources will need to be spent in different ways to end AIDS as a public health threat across the world. In the Caribbean and sub-Saharan Africa, the largest share of resources is needed for HIV treatment services. By contrast, where epidemics are expanding—in parts of Asia and the Pacific, eastern Europe and central Asia, Latin America, and the Middle East and north Africa—the largest share of HIV resources will be needed for HIV prevention services.

Globally, antiretroviral therapy will account for the largest share of resource needs in 2030, followed closely by primary HIV prevention efforts.

FIGURE 3.4

Resource needs in low- and middle-income countries in 2030 to reach global targets

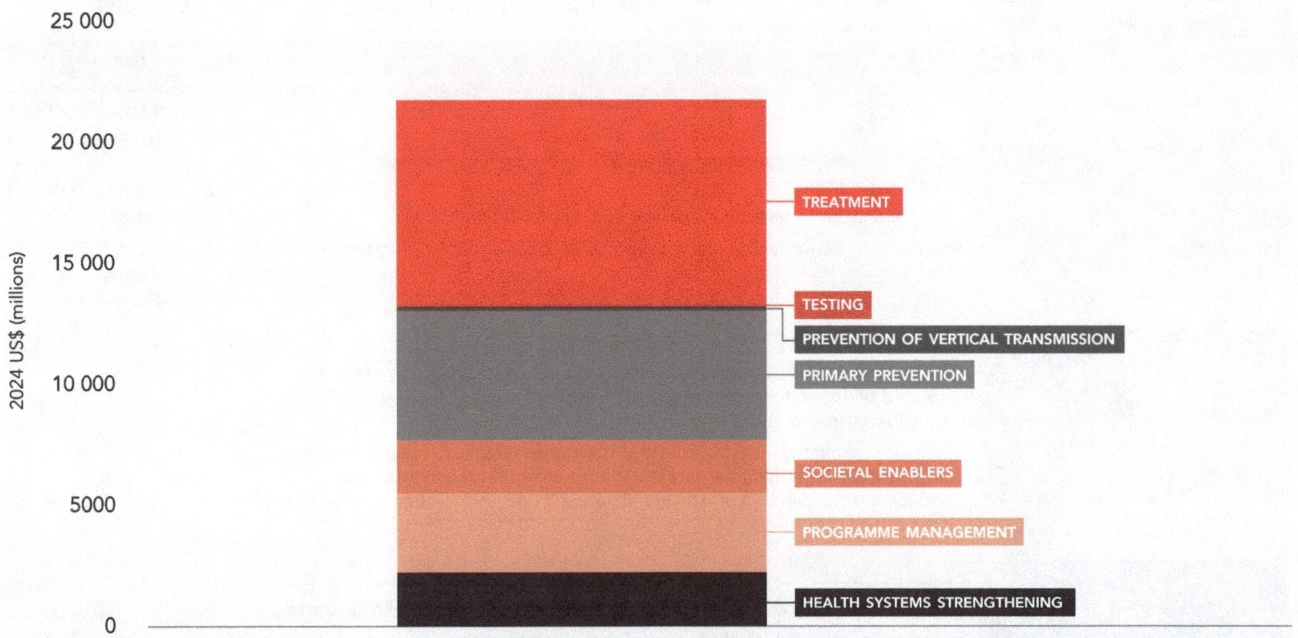

Source: Stover J, Mattur D, Siapka M, Pliakas T, Valladares-Cardona R. The impact and cost of reaching the UNAIDS global HIV targets. medRxiv preprint, 2025.

UNAIDS estimates that it is feasible for the domestic share of HIV financing to rise from 52% in 2024 to two-thirds by 2030. Even if countries are able to reach this benchmark, however, an additional US$ 6 billion annually will need to be mobilized with donor and international funding.

Critical importance of continuing international support for efforts to end AIDS

Although international HIV assistance is expected to continue to decline in future years, hopes for ending AIDS as a public health threat by 2030 depend on maintaining this source of financing as domestic funding for the HIV response increases and ensuring a sound, thoughtful transition to greater country ownership and financing. Sustaining global solidarity in the quest to end AIDS is particularly pivotal for responses in low-income countries, for programmatic elements of the response that have relied heavily on donor support, and for preserving and further strengthening community-led responses, including for key and priority populations.

Developments in the second half of 2025—with respect to the two primary funders of global HIV programmes, the Global Fund and PEPFAR—provide opportunities for countries to invest in programmes and reach the people who need services the most. This can only be achieved when communities of people living with, affected by or at risk of HIV are engaged in developing those programmes.

Renewed donor support with the America First Global Health Strategy and pledges to the Global Fund replenishment in the amount of USD 11.34 billion—with more countries still to make pledges provide opportunities for countries to invest in programmes to reach the people who need services the most.

In September 2025, the United States Government released the America First Global Health Strategy *(9)*. This reaffirms the commitment of the Government to work with countries to achieve the 95–95–95 targets and support the broader goal of ending AIDS as a public health threat. Beginning with bridge funding from October 2025 through March 2026, the United States Government has committed to maintaining 100% of funding for all frontline commodities (including HIV test kits and antiretroviral medicines) and to pay the salaries of the frontline health workers (primarily nurses and community health workers) currently covered by PEPFAR, while co-investment increases. The Strategy also commits to ensuring data systems are in place for accountability and to monitor epidemiological trends, service delivery and supply chains.

By the end of 2025, the United States aims to have negotiated multiyear bilateral agreements with the 71 countries that currently receive United States health assistance. The multiyear agreements will include expectations for greater domestic co-investment in HIV programmes, with further United States support predicated on countries' achievement of co-investment milestones.

There is also encouraging evidence of continued international support for the Global Fund. Co-hosted by South Africa and the United Kingdom of Great Britain and Northern Ireland, the Global Fund's eighth replenishment offered an opportunity for several countries *(95)* and many organizations such as foundations and industries to further contribute to the global HIV response.

The Global Fund is a lead funder in efforts to promote the long-term sustainability of national HIV responses. In its updated policy on sustainability, transition and co-financing, the Global Fund pledges to support early and timely transition planning by countries currently receiving Global Fund assistance in line with UNAIDS sustainability roadmaps (96). The policy requires that recipients of Global Fund support to meet co-financing requirements and increase their co-financing over each allocation period. Countries that graduate to upper-middle-income status become ineligible for Global Fund HIV support unless they can demonstrate a high burden of HIV.

Philanthropic foundations contribute US$ 450 million–550 million each year to the HIV response in low- and middle-income countries. These contributions—driven by key partners such as the Ford Foundation, the Gates Foundation and the Wellcome Trust—form a vital pillar of international HIV financing, complementing bilateral and multilateral donors and domestic investments. The Gates Foundation announcement that it intends to accelerate its giving over the next two decades offers hope that philanthropic contributions to the HIV response might increase even further in future years (97).

Following agreement by Health Ministers from the world's largest economies at G20 meetings in 2024, Brazil has assembled a Global Coalition to achieve more equitable access to health technologies by building local and regional capacities to develop and produce innovative vaccines, medicines and diagnostics (98). South Africa's presidency of the G20 in 2025 featured the work of an independent panel of experts that has called on world leaders to address a global inequality crisis that is fuelling political and economic instability, slowing the AIDS response and making the world more vulnerable to future pandemics (99).

Sustaining and rebuilding HIV-related official development assistance is only one of many ways that high-income countries can mobilize resources towards ending AIDS as a public health threat. Donor countries can also use their leverage to support debt relief (including debt-to-health swaps) and increased concessional funding by multilateral development banks (100). By intervening to de-risk investments in health services in low- and middle-income countries, donor countries can help shape markets and encourage private-sector health investments. As holders of the largest share of Special Drawing Rights of the International Monetary Fund, donors have the ability to reallocate their Special Drawing Rights to expand access of low- and middle-income countries to hard currency for investing in HIV and other health programmes (101).

Country-led efforts to ensure long-term sustainability of the HIV response

Continuing and amplifying recent momentum towards increased domestic financing will be pivotal to ending AIDS as a public health threat by 2030. In this regard, processes for development of HIV response sustainability roadmaps in more than 30 countries are a promising sign.

Bolstering national taxation systems offers one avenue for mobilizing new resources for HIV and other health investments. For example, Uganda's sustainability roadmap aims to increase domestic tax collection to 20% of gross domestic product (from 14% currently) by 2030. In 2025, WHO launched a major global effort for countries to raise US$ 1 trillion in new funding over the coming decade through imposition and earmarking of taxes on tobacco, alcohol and sugary beverages *(102)*.

Relieving national debt burdens is needed to open up domestic fiscal space in many low- and middle-income countries. The Global Fund has facilitated debt-to-health swaps for at least 11 low- and middle-income countries with Australia, Germany and Spain, mobilizing US$ 330 million for new health investments *(103)*.

As part of the global push to achieve universal health coverage, many low- and middle-income countries have either implemented or are implementing national health insurance schemes that have the potential to absorb costs to cover HIV-related services. Among the first 12 HIV response sustainability roadmaps, six prioritized integrating HIV-related services into health insurance benefit packages.

An openness to innovative financing approaches is evident in a number of HIV response sustainability roadmaps. Zimbabwe, for example, aims to explore options such as "development bonds, blended finance, funding from non-traditional donors, capital development funds portion to health, and corporate social responsibility funds" *(104)*.

National sustainability roadmaps highlight the importance of strengthening country capacity to manage how HIV resources are used and improve the efficiency of HIV spending. Zimbabwe calls for actions to "strengthen public financial management systems for health and HIV to enable more accurate, transparent and needs-based budget planning at a national and sub-national level" *(104)*.

Providing community-led responses with the resources they need

The Global AIDS Strategy 2026–2031 outlines strategic action steps to ensure community leadership is recognized, nurtured and adequately supported. Designated community representatives should be engaged in all decision-making levels of the response, including the development of policy guidance, targets and accountability frameworks. Laws, policies and regulations that limit the ability of community-led organizations to participate fully as leaders of the response must be removed or reformed.

Governments, donors and other stakeholders must ensure all facets of community-led responses are adequately supported, with minimum thresholds for domestic allocations for community-led service delivery established to ensure consistency and equity in financial support. To promote the sustainability of community-led service delivery systems, communities must be provided with digital tools, campaigns and key population- or youth-friendly drop-in centres. In addition to support for community-delivered services, community-led responses should be enabled to play their unique role in addressing societal enablers, including through platforms such as Education-Plus. Community-led monitoring and resources must be adequately resourced and taken into account in planning and decision-making processes. Countries should also prioritize support for capacity-strengthening, resilience and preparedness of community-led organizations.

Cultivating and optimizing partnerships

National and subnational governments must lead on efforts to mobilize the resources needed to end AIDS as a public health threat, but they do not need to act alone. Services are primarily provided at the local level. It is also often at this level where new productive partnerships have been developed with the private sector, philanthropies, faith-based organizations, civil society and others. These partnerships between communities, local authorities and the wider community at local level are critical for the success of the HIV response

In many countries, faith-based organizations provide a substantial share of health services delivery *(9, 105)*. The new America First Global Health Strategy prioritizes working with faith-based organizations, citing the community programme of Circle of Hope Zambia, which has been scaled to seven of the 10 provinces in Zambia and has achieved 95% viral suppression among people receiving its services *(9)*.

Seven of the 12 earliest HIV response sustainability roadmaps call for greater engagement of the private sector in the financing and delivery of integrated HIV services. Uganda, for example, aims to ensure 25% of service delivery for health and related non-health services involve the private sector *(72)*, and Zambia aims to promote public–private partnership models for HIV services *(75)*. The Rwandan government has partnered with Microsoft and others to strengthen data management and interoperability *(106)*.

Harnessing innovation to magnify impact and optimize efficiency

Innovations have the potential to make finite resources go further and maximize the public health impact of HIV investments.

LONG-ACTING INJECTABLE ANTIRETROVIRAL MEDICINES

In recent years, the emergence of long-acting injectable PrEP regimens as a complement to daily oral PrEP has energized the HIV response. Providing 2 million person-years of twice-yearly injectable PrEP to people from populations facing the highest HIV incidence could avert 50 000 new HIV infections over three years *(107)*.

Momentum for uptake of long-acting antiretroviral medicines increased in 2025, with WHO issuing new guidelines in July 2025 *(108)*. In September 2025, the United States Government announced that PEPFAR would support efforts by the Global Fund to provide long-acting PrEP to up to 2 million people in high-burden settings *(109)*. The Gates Foundation announced a partnership with Indian generic manufacturer Hetero Labs to manufacture generic versions of long-acting PrEP at a cost of US$ 40 per person per year, with the aim of making the intervention affordable to national health systems *(110)*. CHAI and Unitaid entered into a similar partnership with Dr. Reddy's Laboratories to manufacture generic long-acting PrEP at the same annual price of $US 40 *(111)*.

Communities play a critical role to create demand for health products by organizing people living with or affected by HIV into networks and by holding donors, governments and multilateral agencies accountable. When new technologies such as long-acting PrEP are developed, community-led organizations work to build demand and deliver services in acceptable and accessible ways *(112, 113)*. Especially in a context of political hesitation and funding setbacks, strengthened community-led responses are an opportunity to continue transforming the HIV response from a top-down model to one rooted in solidarity, dignity, resilience, human rights and gender equality.

DIGITAL INNOVATIONS, INCLUDING ARTIFICIAL INTELLIGENCE

Digital innovations offer opportunities for low- and middle-income countries to leapfrog many of the developmental stages other countries have experienced in managing health information and health systems. Digital tools for health care include electronic medical records; telehealth, mobile health and other digital service delivery innovations; and data visualization and other methods to enable timely, strategic decision-making on health policy and programmes. The HIV response has played a key role in helping countries incorporate digital health tools, with the Global Fund and PEPFAR providing critical support for integrated health information systems and digital health-care tools *(114)*.

HIV sustainability roadmaps prioritize improved management and use of data to enhance the efficiency and impact of national responses. To move towards a "single, unified national health information system", for example, Kenya is prioritizing an assessment and mapping of HIV data tools, electronic medical records and reporting systems nationwide and creation of a national consensus for a "unified, government-owned, interoperable national data ecosystem and infrastructure" *(115)*.

The rapid emergence of artificial intelligence as a pillar of contemporary life presents considerable opportunities to enhance HIV outcomes and optimize the health returns on HIV investments. A systematic review of available evidence in 2025 found that artificial intelligence is already improving the reach and performance of a broad range of HIV treatment and care programmes *(116)*.

For example, artificial intelligence can aid in interpreting images from HIV self-testing kits, improving accuracy and aiding in the linkage of people newly diagnosed with HIV to treatment and care *(117)*. Artificial intelligence can enable the analysis of large datasets to forecast commodity stockouts *(118)*.

Artificial intelligence chatbots hold promise for improving HIV service delivery and uptake. In a PrEP initiative in Nigeria, 90% of study participants engaged with a chatbot, with 56% of users requesting an HIV self-test kit *(119)*. In Zambia, an artificial intelligence chatbot supported the integration of HIV prevention in family planning services, enabling linkage to PrEP *(120)*. A potential advantage of artificial intelligence chatbots in HIV service delivery is that they can provide an excellent outlet for people with sensitive or difficult questions that they might be disinclined to ask another human being. In 2025, UNAIDS and WHO published guidance for budgeting and resource planning for the use of virtual HIV interventions *(121)*.

To fully seize the opportunities and promise of artificial intelligence, several important actions are needed, including steps to ensure digital literacy and access to pertinent technologies, and creating safeguards to ensure tools protect individual privacy, avoid gender bias, and are not used to further stigmatize people from key populations, especially in settings where their behaviours are criminalized. Efforts to roll out artificial intelligence to improve the reach and impact of HIV services require focused resources, actions to shape markets in ways that make artificial intelligence applications affordable and accessible, and clearer guidance, particularly as the field continues to evolve *(118)*.

Moving forward: leveraging a new global AIDS strategy to hasten ending AIDS and build sustainability

The Global AIDS Strategy 2026–2031 provides a clear roadmap to ensure success and long-term sustainability in the decades-long global response to AIDS. Key to ending AIDS as a public health threat will be providing antiretroviral therapy to 40 million people, reaching at least 20 million people with antiretroviral-based prevention methods, and ensuring all HIV-related services are free of stigma and discrimination (Figure 3.5). Reaching the target of 90% of people with viral load suppression will be critical to protecting the health of people living with HIV, prevent advanced HIV disease, co-morbidities (including cryptococcal meningits) and to preventing new HIV infections *(122)*.

FIGURE 3.5

40 + 20 goals: global HIV treatment and prevention targets for 2030

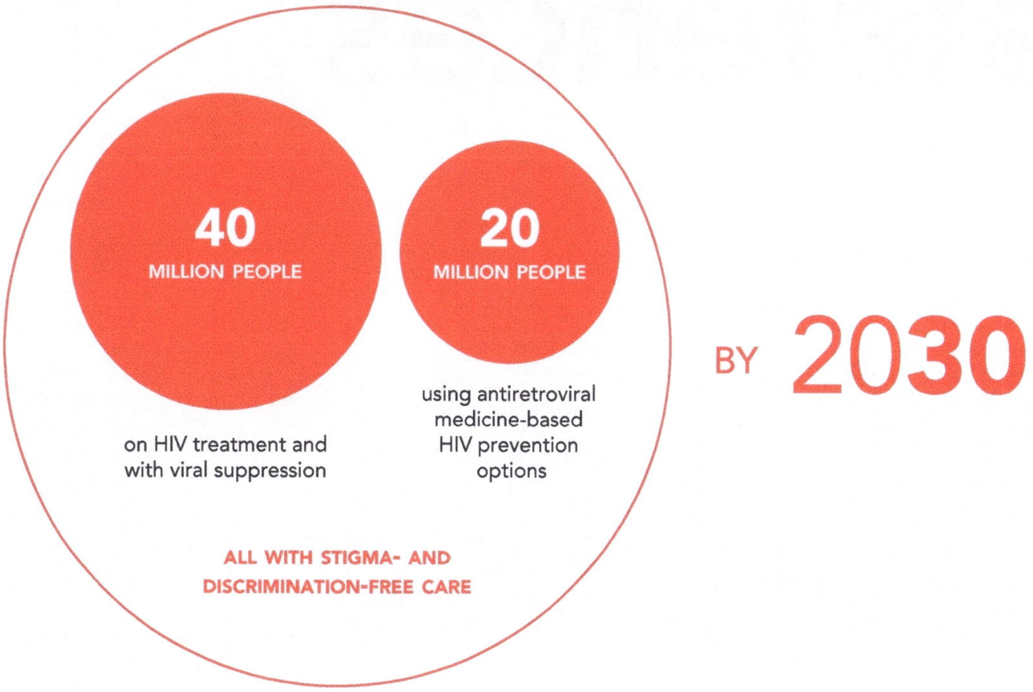

Source: Global AIDS Strategy 2026–2031.

The planned 2026 high-level meeting on HIV and AIDS will afford a global platform for renewing and further strengthening global commitment to end AIDS as a public health threat. The meeting will allow for a review of achievements, persistent gaps and evolving challenges and the forging of a strong global consensus for collective action to reach the 2030 goal.

Although financial resources alone cannot end AIDS as a public health threat, sustained and sufficient funding remains indispensable to achieving the 2023 targets. We call on all partners to renew and strengthen their commitment to closing HIV financial gaps and investing in long-term sustainability.

UNAIDS will continue to support countries in planning for sustainability, including mobilizing essential resources and dismantling obstacles to further progress. The Joint Programme will also continue to support countries in collecting data to monitor progress towards global HIV goals and in holding the global community accountable for their HIV-related commitments.

After decades of delivering results and saving lives, the global HIV response is within reach of its goal to end AIDS as a public health threat and build a sustainable response. HIV programmes are at a time of great vulnerability and risk when people living with, at risk of or affected by HIV are losing access to lifesaving services and the organizations that support those communities are being decimated. There is hope, however, as seen through the political will and the resilience that both communities and countries have demonstrated in the past months. The world has come a very long way already on this journey and now is not the time to pause or step back. Now is the time to keep the promise and end AIDS by 2030.

References

1 WHO issues guidance to address drastic global health financing cuts. Geneva: World Health Organization; 2025 (https://www.who.int/news/item/03-11-2025-who-issues-guidance-to-address-drastic-global-health-financing-cuts).

2 Sullivan PS, Juhasz M, DuBose SN, Le G, Brisco K, Islet D, et al. Association of state-level PrEP coverage and new HIV diagnoses in the USA from 2012 to 2022: an ecological analysis of the population impact of PrEP. Lancet HIV. 2025;12:E440–E448. https://doi.org/10.1016/S2352-3018(25)00036-0.

3 Wexler A, Kates J. Lief E, UNAIDS. Donor government funding for HIV in low- and middle-income countries in 2024. Washington, DC and Geneva: KFF and Joint United Nations Programme on HIV/AIDS; 2025 (https://files.kff.org/attachment/Report-Donor-Government-Funding-for-HIV-in-Low-and-Middle-Income-Countries-in-2024.pdf).

4 Dewast L. Vulnerable South Africans struggle to find HIV medication after U.S. foreign aid cuts. PBS News, 24 August 2025 (https://www.pbs.org/newshour/world/vulnerable-south-africans-struggle-to-find-hiv-medication-after-u-s-foreign-aid-cuts).

5 At a crossroads: responding to a new AIDS emergency in Mozambique. Cape Town: Frontline AIDS. Pre-publication, 1 December 2025.

6 Hanging in the balance: the impact of international donor funding cuts on the health, rights and futures of adolescent girls and young women in Africa—a rapid assessment. ATHENA Network; 2025 (https://networkathena.org/hanging-in-the-balance/).

7 Aid cuts are devastating health services in Africa. The Economist, 30 October 2025 (https://www.economist.com/middle-east-and-africa/2025/10/30/aid-cuts-are-devastating-health-services-in-africa?utm_medium=cpc.adword.pd&utm_source=google&ppccampaignID=18156330227&ppcadID=&utm_campaign=a.22brand_pmax&utm_content=conversion.direct-response.anonymous&gclsrc=aw.ds&gad_source=1&gad_campaignid=18156330848&gclid=EAIaIQobChMIybm_ycnxkAMVq5BQBh3H0R7KEAAYASAAEgKu5fD_BwE).

8 Projected transitions from Global Fund country allocations by 2028: projections by component. Geneva: Global Fund to Fight AIDS, Tuberculosis and Malaria; 2024 (https://www.theglobalfund.org/media/13893/cr_projected-transitions-2028_list_en.pdf).

9 America First Global Health Strategy. Washington, DC: United States Department of State; 2025 (https://www.state.gov/wp-content/uploads/2025/09/America-First-Global-Health-Strategy-Report.pdf).

10 Matse S, Dlamini T, Nyapokoto C. Adapting for impact: funding shifts and HIV programme realignment in Eswatini, Kingdom of Eswatini, Ministry of Health. Presented at the CQUIN 9th Annual Meeting, 17–21 November 2025, Durban, South Africa.

11 Impact of PEPFAR stop work orders on PrEP. New York: AIDS Vaccine Alliance; 2025 (https://www.prepwatch.org/pepfar-stop-work/).

12 Can't stop. Won't stop. Cape Town: Mothers2Mothers (https://m2m.org/wont-stop/).

13 Mosikare O. Botswana faces new HIV scare as shortage of medicines deepens. Mail & Guardian, 20 October 2025 (https://mg.co.za/africa/2025-10-20-botswana-faces-new-hiv-scare-as-shortage-of-medicines-deepens/).

14 Voluntary medical male circumcision for HIV prevention. Geneva: World Health Organization (https://www.who.int/teams/global-hiv-hepatitis-and-stis-programmes/hiv/prevention/voluntary-medical-male-circumcision).

15 Davis SM, Fellows I, de Leon O, Bastani P, Hakin AJ, Toledo C, et al. Circumcision for HIV prevention in men who have sex with men: an updated meta-analysis. MedRxiv preprint, 2025. https://doi.org/10.1101/2025.07.02.25330772.

16 Brangham W, Raskin MK. How USAID cuts are impacting the fight against HIV/AIDS in Kenya. PBS News, 12 June 2025 (https://www.pbs.org/newshour/show/how-usaid-cuts-are-impacting-the-fight-against-hiv-in-kenya).

17 Abandoned in crisis: the impact of U.S. global health funding cuts in Democratic Republic of the Congo (DRC). New York: Physicians for Human Rights; 2025 (https://phr.org/wp-content/uploads/2025/07/PHR-Research-Brief-Aid-Cuts-DRC-2025.pdf).

18 Shuttered clinics, preventable deaths: the impact of U.S. global health funding cuts in Ethiopia. New York: Physicians for Human Rights; 2025 (https://phr.org/wp-content/uploads/2025/06/PHR-Ethiopia-Research-Brief-June-2025.pdf).

19 Stevens O, Sabin K, Anderson RL, Garcia SA, Willis K, Rao A, et al. Population size, HIV prevalence, and antiretroviral therapy coverage among key populations in sub-Saharan Africa: a collection and synthesis of survey data, 2010–23. Lancet Glob Health. 2024;12:e1400–e1412. https://doi.org/10.1016/S2214-109X(24)00236-5.

20 How HIV funding cuts are undermining years of progress in Zimbabwe. New York: Médecins sans Frontières; 2025 (https://www.doctorswithoutborders.org/latest/how-hiv-funding-cuts-are-undermining-years-progress-zimbabwe).

21 Tracking the freeze: real-time impact on key populations. Global Black Gay Men Connect; 2025 (https://gbgmc.org/impact-us-funding-cuts/#country-impact).

22 The human costs of policy shifts: the fallout of United States' foreign aid cuts on harm reduction programming and people who use drugs. Downham Market, United Kingdom: International Network of People Who Use Drugs; 2025 (https://inpud.net/wp-content/uploads/2025/04/The-Human-Cost-of-Policy-Shifts-Rapid-Assessment-Findings.pdf).

23 Policy guidance by HIV intervention area. Geneva: World Health Organization (https://www.who.int/europe/teams/joint-infectious-diseases-unit-(jid)/hiv-aids#:~:text=Harm%20reduct).

24 Walimbwa Wambaya J, Ligare F, Wanjiku J, Mwendwa K, Ouma K, Digolo V, et al. The consequences of dismantling community-led HIV programming in Kenya: a call to action from the HEKA programme research partnership in Kenya. BMJ Glob Health. 2025;10:e019502. https://doi.org/10.1136/bmjgh-2025-019502.

25 HIV market impact memo. Boston, MA: Clinton Health Access Initiative; 2025 (https://www.clintonhealthaccess.org/wp-content/uploads/2025/07/2025-Q2-CHAI-HIV-Market-Impact-Memo.pdf).

26 South Africa state of health. Johannesburg: Ritshidze; 2025 (https://ritshidze.org.za/wp-content/uploads/2025/10/Ritshidze-National-State-of-Health-October-2025.pdf).

27 Tantum LK, Anderson DM, Halwiindi H, Herce M, Mbizvo MT, et al. The impacts of United States foreign development assistance reductions on health system building blocks at healthcare facilities in Zambia: a mixed-methods study. MedRxiv preprint, 2025. https://doi.org/10.1101/2025.10.06.25337414.

28 Kachingwe E, Mutanda N, Ntjikelane V, Benade M, Manganye M, Malala L, et al. Characteristics and six-month viral load suppression of clients presenting with advanced HIV disease in South Africa. PLOS Glob Public Health. 2025;5:e0004927. https://doi.org/10.1371/journal.pgph.0004927.

29 Pita TP, Misra S, Madonsela T, Tshazi A, Bosman S, Ayakaka I, et al. "When your CD4 count lowers that is when you are similar to a person that is non-existent": a qualitative exploration of perceptions around advanced HIV disease. BMC Public Health. 2025;25:2325. https://doi.org/10.1186/s12889-025-23588-1.

30 "The system is folding in on itself": the impact of U.S. global health funding cuts in Kenya. New York: Physicians for Human Rights; 2025 (https://phr.org/wp-content/uploads/2025/07/PHR-Research-Brief-Aid-Cuts-Kenya-2025.pdf).

31 On the brink of catastrophe: U.S. foreign aid disruptions to HIV services in Tanzania and Uganda. New York: Physicians for Human Rights; 2025 (https://phr.org/wp-content/uploads/2025/09/On-the-Brink-of-Catastrophe-U.S.-Foreign-Aid-Disruption-to-HIV-Services-in-Tanzania-and-Uganda_PHR_September-2025.pdf).

32 Impact of community-led and community-based HIV service delivery beyond HIV: case studies from eastern and southern Africa. Geneva: Joint United Nations Programme on HIV/AIDS; 2025 (https://www.unaids.org/sites/default/files/media_asset/jc3129_community-service-delivery-impact-beyond-hiv_en.pdf?utm_source=chatgpt.com).

33 Impact of US funding cuts on HIV programmes in east and southern Africa: 15 March–1 April. Geneva: Joint United Nations Programme on HIV/AIDS; 2025 (https://www.unaids.org/sites/default/files/2025-04/20250401_ESA_SITREP.pdf).

34 No more business as usual: a gender-transformative response to the USAID freeze crisis is urgent. International Community of Women Living with HIV; 2025 (https://www.wlhiv.org/post/no-more-business-as-usual-report).

35 An urgent call to support youth-led organizations. Geneva: Joint United Nations Programme on HIV/AIDS; 2025 (https://www.unaids.org/en/resources/presscentre/featurestories/2025/may/20250528_youth).

36 Take the rights path: World AIDS Day report 2024. Geneva: Joint United Nations Programme on HIV/AIDS; 2024 (https://www.unaids.org/sites/default/files/media_asset/take-the-rights-path-to-end-aids_en.pdf).

37 Beyrer C, Kamarulzaman A, Isbell M, Amon J, Baral S, Bassett MT, et al. Under threat: the International AIDS Society–Lancet Commission on Health and Human Rights. Lancet. 2024;403:1374–1418. https://doi.org/10.1016/S0140-6736(24)00302-7.

38 Anti-gender movements. New York: Global Action for Trans Equality; 2025 (https://gate.ngo/knowledge-portal/initiative/anti-gender-movements).

39 New global data reveals rising HIV criminalisation amid stalling legal reforms. Amsterdam: HIV Justice Network; 2025 (https://www.hivjustice.net/news/new-global-data-reveals-rising-hiv-criminalisation-amid-stalling-legal-reforms/).

40 Criminalization of HIV and sex work in western and central Africa. Montreal and Kinshasa: HIV Legal Network and HODSAS for HIV Justice Worldwide; 2025 (https://www.hivlegalnetwork.ca/site/criminalization-of-hiv-and-sex-work-in-western-and-central-africa).

41 People under attack 2024. Johannesburg: CIVICUS (https://monitor.civicus.org/globalfindings_2024/).

42 AIDS, crisis and the power to transform: UNAIDS global AIDS update 2025. Geneva: Joint United Nations Programme on HIV/AIDS; 2025 (https://www.unaids.org/sites/default/files/2025-07/2025-global-aids-update-JC3153_en.pdf).

43 Breaking the inequality–pandemic cycle: building true health security: findings and recommendations of the Global Council. Geneva: Global Council on Inequality, AIDS and Pandemics; 2025 (https://www.unaids.org/sites/default/files/2025-11/2025_global-council-inequality-report_en.pdf).

44 Revenue statistics in Africa 2024. Paris: Organisation for Economic Co-operation and Development; 2024 (https://www.oecd.org/en/publications/revenue-statistics-in-africa-2024_78e9af3a-en/full-report.html).

45 Global humanitarian overview 2025. New York: United Nations Office for the Coordination of Humanitarian Affairs; 2025 (https://www.unocha.org/publications/report/world/global-humanitarian-overview-2025-enarfres).

46 Adaptation gap report 2023. Nairobi: United Nations Environment Programme; 2023 (https://www.unep.org/resources/adaptation-gap-report-2023).

47 HIV response sustainability primer. Geneva: Joint United Nations Programme on HIV/AIDS; 2024 (https://www.unaids.org/en/resources/documents/2024/20240117_HIV_response_sustainability).

48 African Union (AU) roadmap to 2030 and beyond: sustaining the AIDS response, ensuring systems strengthening and health security for the development of Africa. Addis Ababa: African Union; 2025 (https://au.int/sites/default/files/documents/44542-doc-AU_Roadmap_to_2030._EN.pdf).

49 Africa's health financing in a new era—April, 2025. Addis Ababa: Africa Centers for Disease Control and Prevention; 2025 (https://africacdc.org/news-item/africas-health-financing-in-a-new-era-april-2025/).

50 Jerving S. African Union finally approves framework for Africa CDC epidemics fund. Devex, 21 February 2025 (https://www.devex.com/news/african-union-finally-approves-framework-for-africa-cdc-epidemics-fund-109456).

51 Jerving S. The "Accra reset": time's up for the legacy aid system. Devex, 1 October 2025 (https://www.devex.com/news/the-accra-reset-time-s-up-for-the-legacy-aid-system-110845).

52 Decision on the Extraordinary Summit on Ending Aids by 2030 and Addressing Preventable Maternal Deaths, Communicable and Non-Communicable Diseases Endemic African Union (AU) Roadmap to 2030 and beyond: sustaining the aids response, ensuring systems strengthening and health security for the development of Africa. Addis Ababa: African Union; 2025 (https://africanlii.org/en/akn/aa-au/doc/decision/2025-02-16/908/eng).

53 55 AFR/RC/74/6. Framework for strengthening local production of medicines, vaccines, and other health technologies in the WHO African region 2025–2035. 74th session of the WHO Regional Committee for Africa, Brazzaville, 2024 (https://www.afro.who.int/sites/default/files/2024-07/AFR-RC74-6%20Framework%20for%20strengthening%20local%20production%20of%20medicines,%20vaccines%20and%20other%20health%20technologies%20in%20the%20WHO%20African%20Region.pdf).

54 Nakola S. New Africa CDC platform boosts regional health manufacturing. China Daily, 14 October 2025 (https://www.chinadaily.com.cn/a/202510/14/WS68ee3e6ca310f735438b4f32.html).

55 2nd EAC Regional Pharmaceutical Manufacturing Plan of Action 2017–2018. Arusha: Eastern African Community (https://industrialization.go.ke/sites/default/files/2023-08/2nd%20EAC%20Regional%20Pharmaceutical%20Manufacturing%20Plan%20of%20Action%2020172027.pdf).

56 African Vaccine Manufacturing Accelerator (AVMA). Geneva: Global Alliance for Vaccines and Immunization; 2025 (https://www.gavi.org/programmes-impact/types-support/regional-manufacturing-strategy/avma).

57 African pooled procurement mechanism (APPM). Addis Ababa: African Centers for Disease Control and Prevention (https://africacdc.org/appm/).

58 Steuerwald T, Blair D, Cowan E, Isbell M, Boova S, Firmat J, et al. Improving the efficiency of the regulatory approvals of HIV in vitro diagnostics in low- and middle-income countries: perspective of the IAS Industry Liaison Forum diagnostic partners. PLOS Glob Public Health. 2025;5:e0004169. https://doi.org/10.1371/journal.pgph.0004169.

59 ASEAN leaders' declaration on ending inequalities and getting on track to end AIDS by 2030. Jakarta: Association of Southeast Asian Nations; 2022 (https://asean.org/wp-content/uploads/2022/11/36-ASEAN-Leaders-Declaration-on-Ending-Inequalities-and-Getting-on-Track-to-End-AIDS-by-2030.pdf).

60 Regional action framework for health financing to achieve universal health coverage and sustainable development in the Western Pacific. Manila: World Health Organization Regional Office for the Western Pacific; 2025 (https://www.who.int/publications/i/item/9789290620976).

61 CARICOM DSG affirms support for closing gaps and accelerating progress for HIV prevention and care. Georgetown, Guyana: CARICOM Secretariat; 2025 (https://caricom.org/caricom-dsg-affirms-support-for-closing-gaps-and-accelerating-progress-for-hiv-prevention-and-care/).

62 Adejoro L. Nigeria allocated additional $200 m to health in 2025 budget—WHO. Healthwise, 13 April 2025 (https://healthwise.punchng.com/nigeria-allocated-additional-200m-to-health-in-2025-budget-who/).

63 Mugenyi H. Uganda increases health sector budget to Shs 5.87 tn in FY 2025/26. NilePost, 12 June 2025 (https://nilepost.co.ug/health/264596/uganda-increases-health-sector-budget-to-shs-587-tn-in-fy-202526).

64 UNAIDS commends Côte d'Ivoire's commitment to increase domestic funding for HIV. Geneva: Joint United Nations Programme on HIV/AIDS; 2025 (https://www.unaids.org/en/resources/presscentre/pressreleaseandstatementarchive/2025/july/20250724_cotedivoire).

65 Cohen J. Countries to budget more for HIV/AIDS measures as U.S. withdraws aid. Science, 14 July 2025 (https://www.science.org/content/article/countries-budget-more-hiv-aids-measures-u-s-withdraws-aid#:~:text=Many%20eyes%20are%20on%20how,%2C%20corporations%2C%20and%20other%20donors).

66 Christopher J. Tanzania targets Sh 586.5 billion from new domestic taxes to bridge HIV and health funding gap. The Citizen, 12 June (https://www.thecitizen.co.tz/tanzania/news/national/tanzania-targets-sh586-4-billion-from-new-domestic-taxes-to-bridge-hiv-and-health-funding-gap-5078984).

67 Ochanda RM, Mwangomale A, Banda A, Ngwenya A, Macwilliam J, Chikanya W, et al. Domestic resource mobilization for HIV in Africa: a comparative analysis of country policies and practices. Abstract OAE0202. Presented at the 13th International AIDS Society Conference on HIV Science, Kigali, 2025.

68 Impact of US funding cuts on HIV programmes in Guatemala UNAIDS. Geneva: Joint United Nations Programme on HIV/AIDS; 2025 (https://www.unaids.org/en/resources/presscentre/featurestories/2025/march/20250314_Guatemala_fs).

69 Impact of US funding cuts on HIV programmes in Viet Nam. Geneva: Joint United Nations Programme on HIV/AIDS; 2025 (https://www.unaids.org/en/resources/presscentre/featurestories/2025/march/20250319_VietNam_fs).

70 HIV sustainability planning: analytical resource: Kenya. Geneva: Joint United Nations Programme on HIV/AIDS; 2024 (https://sustainability.unaids.org/wp-content/uploads/2024/08/Kenya__-Executive-Summary-May-2024.pdf).

71 HIV response sustainability primer. Geneva: Joint United Nations Programme on HIV/AIDS; 2024 (https://www.unaids.org/sites/default/files/media_asset/HIV%20response%20sustainability%20response%20primer_web.pdf).

72 Uganda's roadmap to end HIV and TB as a public health threat by 2030: part A. Kampala: Uganda's AIDS Commission; 2025.

73 Feuille de route pour la durabilité de la riposte au VIH au Togo: partie A. Lomé: Conseil national de lutte contre le Sida et les infections sexuellement transmissible, Republique Togolaise; 2024 (https://sustainability.unaids.org/wp-content/uploads/2024/06/Feuille_-de_route_Durabilite_Togo_Vesion-valide-GT.pdf).

74 HIV response sustainability roadmap for Malawi. Lilongwe: Government of Malawi; 2025 (https://sustainability.unaids.org/wp-content/uploads/2024/06/Malawi_SRM_PartA.pdf).

75 Zambia HIV response sustainability roadmap: Vision 2030 and beyond—part 1. Lusaka: Zambia Ministry of Health (https://sustainability.unaids.org/wp-content/uploads/2024/06/Zambia_SRM_A.pdf).

76 HIV and TB sustainability roadmap for the Kingdom of Lesotho towards 2030 and beyond. Maseru: Lesotho National AIDS Commission; 2024 (https://sustainability.unaids.org/wp-content/uploads/2024/06/Lesotho_SRM_A.pdf).

77 National HIV response sustainability assessment and roadmap (part A). Accra: Office of the President of Ghana; 2025 (https://sustainability.unaids.org/wp-content/uploads/2024/06/GHANA-HIV-SUSTAINABILITY-ROADMAP-PART_-A-FINAL-Version-GAC-AND-UNAIDS_.pdf).

78 HIV sustainability planning: analytical resource: Nigeria. Geneva: Joint United Nations Programme on HIV/AIDS; 2024 (https://sustainability.unaids.org/wp-content/uploads/2024/08/Nigeria__-Executive-Summary-May-2024.pdf).

79 Okorie K. As US terminates funding, Nigeria shifts focus to sustain HIV progress. Health Policy Watch, 28 February 2025 (https://healthpolicy-watch.news/as-us-terminates-funding-nigeria-shifts-focus-to-sustain-hiv-progress).

80 2024 annual report. Harare: GALZ; 2024 (https://www.galz.org/_files/ugd/241bc6_83cffb99b0be448aa417503e306e8759.pdf).

81 Kisika S. Kenyan, Ugandan groups demand inclusive HIV programs to fill US funding gap. Washington Blade, 28 July 2025 (https://www.washingtonblade.com/2025/07/28/kenyan-ugandan-groups-demand-inclusive-hiv-programs-to-fi).

82 Integrated person-centred health services: translating learnings from the HIV response to pave the way to universal health coverage. Washington, DC: Friends of the Global Fight Against AIDS, Tuberculosis and Malaria, JSI and PATH; 2023 (https://www.theglobalfight.org/wp-content/uploads/2023/10/Integrated-Person-Centered-Health-Services-Translating-Learnings-from-the-HIV-Response-to-Pave-the-way-to-UHC.pdf).

83 Bulstra CA, Hontelez JAC, Otto M, Stepanova A, Lamontagne E, Yakusik A, et al. Integrating HIV services and other health services: a systematic review and meta-analysis. PLoS Med. 2021;18:e1003836. https://doi.org/10.1371/journal.pmed.1003836.

84 Ninsiima M, Nyabigambo A, Kagaayi J. Acceptability of integration of cervical cancer screening into routine HIV care, associated factors and perceptions among HIV-infected women: a mixed methods study at Mbarara Regional Referral Hospital, Uganda. BMC Health Serv Res. 2023;23(1):333. https://doi.org/10.1186/s12913-023-09326-6.

85 Global tuberculosis report 2025. Geneva: World Health Organization; 2025 (https://iris.who.int/server/api/core/bitstreams/e97dd6f4-b567-4396-8680-717bac6869a9/content).

86 Chang D, Esber AL, Dear NF, Iroezindu M, Bahemana E, Kibuuka E, et al. Non-communicable diseases by age strata in people living with and without HIV in four African countries. J Int AIDS Soc. 2022;25(Suppl. 4):e25985. https://doi.org/10.1002/jia2.25985.

87 Whitehead S. People with HIV are aging, and the challenges are piling up. NPR, 15 June 2024 (https://www.npr.org/sections/shots-health-news/2024/06/15/nx-s1-4990795/hiv-aids-aging-health-risks-).

88 WHO guideline on HIV service delivery: updated guidance on the integration of diabetes, hypertension and mental health services, and interventions to support adherence to antiretroviral therapy. Geneva: World Health Organization; 2025 (https://iris.who.int/server/api/core/bitstreams/f6e902a0-b37b-4340-8296-39d91f3321bb/content).

89 HIV response sustainability roadmap part A. Dodoma: United Republic of Tanzania Prime Minister's Office; 2024 (https://sustainability.unaids.org/wp-content/uploads/2024/06/Tanzania_SMR_A-.pdf).

90 Roadmap towards the sustainability of HIV, viral hepatitis, tuberculosis and malaria control in Namibia. Windhoek: Namibia Ministry of Health and Social Services; 2024 (https://sustainability.unaids.org/wp-content/uploads/2024/06/Namibia_SRMA.pdf).

91 Ensuring quality health care by reducing HIV-related stigma and discrimination. Geneva: World Health Organization; 2024 (https://www.who.int/publications/i/item/9789240097414).

92 People Living with HIV Stigma Index 2.0: global report 2023. Hear us out: community measuring HIV-related stigma and discrimination. Amsterdam: Global Network of People living with HIV; 2023 (https://development.stigmaindex.org/wp-content/uploads/2023/11/PLHIV-Stigma-Index-Global-Report-2023-3.pdf).

93 Callender D, McManus H, Gray RT, Grulich AE, Carr A, Hoy J, et al. HIV treatment-as-prevention and its effect on incidence of HIV among cisgender gay, bisexual, and other men who have sex with men in Australia: a 10-year longitudinal cohort study. Lancet HIV. 2023;10:E385–E393. https://doi.org/10.1016/S2352-3018(23)00112-1.

94 Germany's commitment to the Global Fund replenishment: a timely investment in health, equity and resilience. Geneva: Global Fund to Fight AIDS, Tuberculosis and Malaria; 2025 (https://www.theglobalfund.org/en/news/2025/2025-10-12-germany-commitment-global-fund-replenishment-timely-investment-health-equity-resilience/).

95 The Global Fund sustainability, transition, and co-financing policy. Geneva: Global Fund to Fight AIDS, Tuberculosis and Malaria; 2024 (https://resources.theglobalfund.org/media/14383/core_sustainability-transition-cofinancing_policy_en.pdf).

96 Gates Foundation will double spending over the next 20 years to accelerate progress on saving and improving lives. Seattle: Gates Foundation; 2025 (https://www.gatesfoundation.org/ideas/media-center/press-releases/2025/05/25th-anniversary-announcement).

97 Rio de Janeiro declaration of the G20 health ministers. Rio de Janeiro: G20 Brasil 2024; 2024 (https://www.unaids.org/en/resources/presscentre/pressreleaseandstatementarchive/2024/november/20241101_g20).

98 G20 global inequality report: full and summary. Pretoria: South African Government (https://www.gov.za/documents/other/g20-global-inequality-report-full-and-summary-04-nov-2025).

99 Germany's commitment to the Global Fund replenishment: a timely investment in health, equity and resilience. Geneva: Global Fund to Fight AIDS, Tuberculosis and Malaria; 2025 (https://www.theglobalfund.org/en/news/2025/2025-10-12-germany-commitment-global-fund-replenishment-timely-investment-health-equity-resilience/).

100 Expanding global health finance: convening report and agenda for action. Washington, DC: Friends of the Global Fight Against AIDS, Tuberculosis and Malaria, ONE Campaign and Results; 2025 (https://www.theglobalfight.org/wp-content/uploads/2025/09/25022F-GF-Global-Health-Finance-Report-R5-DIGITAL-09152025.pdf).

101 Policy brief: rechanneling SDRs in a responsible and efficiency way. New York: Lazard; 2022 (https://www.lazard.com/research-insights/rechanneling-imf-special-drawing-rights-in-a-responsible-and-efficient-way/).

102 WHO launched bold push to raise health taxes and save millions of lives. Geneva: World Health Organization; 2025 (https://www.who.int/news/item/02-07-2025-who-launches-bold-push-to-raise-health-taxes-and-save-millions-of-lives).

103 Debt swaps (Debt2Health). Geneva: Global Fund to Fight AIDS, Tuberculosis and Malaria (https://www.theglobalfund.org/en/how-we-raise-funds/innovative-finance/debt-swaps-debt2health/).

104 Roadmaptransformationframework. Harare: Government of Zimbabwe; 2025.

105 Olivier J, Tsimpo C, Gemignani R, Shojo M, Coulombe H, Dimmock F, et al. Understanding the roles of faith-based health-care providers in Africa: review of the evidence with a focus on magnitude, reach, cost, and satisfaction. Lancet. 2015;386:1765–1775. https://doi.org/10.1016/S0140-6736(15)60251-3.

106 Private sector and philanthropy: Microsoft. Geneva: Global Fund to Fight AIDS, Tuberculosis and Malaria (https://www.theglobalfund.org/en/private-sector-and-philanthropy/profiles/microsoft/).

107 What can modelling tell us about the scale-up of lenacapavir for pre-exposure prophylaxis? Geneva: Joint United Nations Programme on HIV/AIDS; 2025 (https://www.unaids.org/sites/default/files/2025-09/JC3154_lenacapavir-modelling_en.pdf).

108 Guidelines on lenacapavir for HIV prevention and testing strategies for long-acting injectable pre-exposure prophylaxis. Geneva: World Health Organization; 2025 (https://iris.who.int/server/api/core/bitstreams/30ec1404-5338-4459-a6f0-a187c85f3ff1/content).

109 PEPFAR commits to distributing breakthrough HIV drug lenacapavir demonstrating American excellence in science and American leadership in HIV prevention. Washington, DC: United States Department of State; 2025 (https://www.state.gov/releases/the-united-states-presidents-emergency-plan-for-aids-relief/2025/09/pepfar-commits-to-distributing-breakthrough-hiv-drug-lenacapavir-demonstrating-american-excellence-in-science-and-american-leadership-in-hiv-prevention).

110 Gates Foundation partners with Indian manufacturer to drive down cost of, accelerate access to groundbreaking HIV prevention tool. Seattle, WA: Gates Foundation; 2025 (https://www.gatesfoundation.org/ideas/media-center/press-releases/2025/09/hiv-prevention-lenacapavir).

111 Unitaid, CHAI, and Witts RHI enter into landmark agreement with Dr. Reddy's to make HIV prevention tool lenacapavir affordable in LMICs. Geneva: Unitaid; 2025 (https://unitaid.org/news-blog/lenacapavir-for-hiv-prevention/).

112 Ayala G, Sprague L, van der Merwe LL, Thomas RM, Chang J, Arreola S, et al. Peer- and community-led responses to HIV: a scoping review. PLoS One. 2021;16(12):e0260555.

113 Nyagah W, Segal K, Feltham J, Ash A, Major J, Masani M. How might we motivate uptake of the dual prevention pill?Findingsfromhuman-centereddesign research with potential end users, male partners, and healthcare providers. Front Reprod Health. 2023;5:1254953. https://doi.org/10.3389/frph.2023.1254953. Erratum in: Front Reprod Health. 2023 Dec 05;5:1341771. https://doi.org/10.3389/frph.2023.1341771.

114 The Global Fund's unique contribution to universal health coverage and stronger health systems: a review of the evidence and future opportunities. Washington, DC: Friends of the Global Fight Against AIDS, Tuberculosis and Malaria; 2023 (https://www.theglobalfight.org/wp-content/uploads/2023/11/231103-UHC-Report_v3-Digital.pdf).

115 Kenya's operational plan for enhancing country readiness to sustain a resilient HIV response beyond 2030. Kenya Ministry of Health; 2024 (https://sustainability.unaids.org/wp-content/uploads/2024/06/Kenya_s-Operational-Plan-for-Enhancing-Country-Readiness-to-Sustain-a-Resilient-Hiv-Response-Beyond-2030-V8.pdf).

116 Ngcobo S, Madela Mntla E, Shock J, Louw M, Mdonambi L, Serite T, et al. Artificial intelligence for HIV care: a global systematic review of current studies and emerging trends. J Int AIDS Soc. 2025;28:e70045. https://doi.org/10.1002/jia2.70045.

117 Roche SD, Ekwunife OI, Mendonca R, Kwach B, Omollo V, Zhang S, et al. Measuring the performance of computer vision artificial intelligence to interpret images of HIV self-testing results. Front Public Health. 2024;12:1334881. https://doi.org/10.3389/fpubh.2024.1334881.

118 Ratevosian J, Reid M, Ni Z, Mendonca R, Eakle R, Johnson C, et al. Reimagining HIV prevention with artificial intelligence. Lancet HIV. 2025;12:E670–E671. https://doi.org/10.1016/S2352-3018(25)00158-4.

119 Mathur S, Eromhonsele AF, Vallarino Z, Savel C, Oche E, Ononye, O et al. "Let's chat!" Piloting a digital chatbot for HIV prevention among cisgender women and transgender men in Nigeria. AIDS Care. 2025;37:1015–1025. https://doi.org/10.1080/09540121.2025.2470318.

120 Yam EA, Namukonda E, McClair T, Souidi S, Chelwa N, Muntalima N, et al. Developing and testing a chatbot to integrate HIV education into family planning clinic waiting areas in Lusaka, Zambia. Glob Health Sci Pract. 2022;10:e2100721. https://doi.org/10.9745/GHSP-D-21-00721.

121 Budgeting and resource planning guidance for implementing virtual interventions as part of HIV responses. Geneva: Joint United Nations Programme on HIV/AIDS and World Health Organization; 2025 (https://iris.who.int/server/api/core/bitstreams/6dc8b5cc-426c-4643-96a4-462a05fbdece/content).

122 Jarvis JN, Ehrenkranz P, Lawrence DS. Reducing HIV incidence and mortality: two sides of the same coin in the approach to ending AIDS. Lancet HIV. 2025:S2352-3018(25)00265-6. https://doi.org/10.1016/S2352-3018(25)00265-6.